# 'RACE' AND CHILDBIRTH

## 'RACE', HEALTH AND SOCIAL CARE

*Series editors:*

**Professor Waqar I.U. Ahmad**, Professor of Primary Care Research and Director, Centre for Research in Primary Care, University of Leeds.

**Professor Charles Husband**, Professor of Social Analysis and Director, Ethnicity and Social Policy Research Unit (ESPR), University of Bradford.

Minority ethnic groups now constitute over 5 per cent of the UK population. While research literature has mushroomed on the one hand in race and ethnic relations generally, and on the other in clinical and epidemiological studies of differences in conditions and use of health and social services, there remains a dearth of credible social scientific literature on the health and social care of minority ethnic communities. Social researchers have hitherto largely neglected issues of 'race' and ethnicity, while acknowledging the importance of gender, class and, more recently, (dis)ability in both the construction of and provision for health and social care needs. Consequently the available social science texts on health and social care largely reflect the experiences of the white population and have been criticized for marginalizing minority ethnic people.

This series aims to provide an authoritative source of policy relevant texts which specifically address issues of health and social care in contemporary multi-ethnic Britain. Given the rate of change in the structure of health and social care services, demography and the political context of state welfare there is a need for a critical appraisal of the health and social care needs of, and provision for, the minority ethnic communities in Britain. By the nature of the issues we will address, this series will draw upon a wide range of professional and academic expertise, thus enabling a deliberate and necessary integration of theory and practice in these fields. The books will be inter-disciplinary and written in clear, non-technical language which will appeal to a broad range of students, academic and professional with a common interest in 'race', health and social care.

*Current and forthcoming titles*

Waqar I.U. Ahmad: *Ethnicity, Disability and Caring*
Waqar I.U. Ahmad and Karl Atkin: *'Race' and Community Care*
Elizabeth Anionwu and Karl Atkin: *The Politics of Sickle Cell and Thalassaemia – 20 Years On*
Kate Gerrish, Charles Husband and Jennifer Mackenzie: *Nursing for a Multi-ethnic Society*
Savita Katbamna: *'Race' and Childbirth*
Derek Kirton: *'Race', Ethnicity and Adoption*
Lena Robinson: *'Race', Communication and the Caring Professions*

# 'RACE' AND CHILDBIRTH

**Savita Katbamna**

**Open University Press**
Buckingham · Philadelphia

Open University Press
Celtic Court
22 Ballmoor
Buckingham
MK18 1XW

e-mail: enquiries@openup.co.uk
world wide web: http://www.openup.co.uk

and
325 Chestnut Street
Philadelphia, PA 19106, USA

First Published 2000



A catalogue record of this book is available from the British Library

ISBN 0 335 19946 1 (pb) 0 335 19947 X (hb)

*Library of Congress Cataloging-in-Publication Data*
Katbamna, Savita, 1947–
'Race' and childbirth / Savita Katbamna.
p. cm. – (Race, health, and social care)
Includes bibliographical references and index.
ISBN 0-335-19947-X (hb.). – ISBN 0-335-19946-1 (pb.)
1. Childbirth–Great Britain–Cross-cultural studies. 2. Prenatal care–Great Britain–Cross-cultural studies. 3. Gujaratis (Indic people)–Medical care–Great Britain. 4. Bangladeshis–Medical care–Great Britain. 5. Maternal health services–Great Britain.
I. Title. II. Series.
RG526.K38 2000
362.1'982'00941–dc21 99–30674
CIP

Typeset by Graphicraft Limited, Hong Kong
Printed in Great Britain by Biddles Ltd, Guildford and King's Lynn

*To my husband Chandra*
*and daughters Mira and Kamala*

# Contents

# Acknowledgements

A number of people have inspired me to get started on this book. These include Viv Edwards who has been a constant source of support and generously gave her time to comment on various drafts of the book. I am also indebted to Waqar Ahmad for his advice and helpful editorial comments. I would also like to thank Jacinta Evans and Joan Malherbe at Open University Press, who were patient and helpful.

And finally I would like to thank my husband Chandra for reading and commenting on earlier drafts and for his constant and unstinting support which enabled me to finish this book.

# 1

# Introduction

Pregnancy and childbirth are the most significant events in the life cycles of most women, irrespective of social class, culture and ethnic background. This book is about the experiences of pregnancy and childbirth in Britain of two groups of South Asian women with roots in the Indian subcontinent.

In western industrialized nations, advances in medical technology and the dominant role played by medical professionals have had a major influence in determining trends in childbirth practices. In the process, a biological and social event, traditionally supervised and managed by females, has been transformed into a medical emergency. The inexorable rise in the medicalization and hospitalization of childbirth witnessed in the west has become an important consideration for childbearing women, women's organizations and those who have an academic interest in the subject. This is evident from the large volume of literature within the field of social science and medicine, which has examined the impact of current childbirth practices on women's lives.

To date, much of the research effort has been confined to exploring the experiences of white women. Women from minority ethnic groups, who constitute a substantial part of the female population of childbearing age in Britain, have received relatively little attention in the literature. This lack of interest is particularly striking given that women from minority ethnic groups in Britain are not immune to the vagaries of current childbirth practices as they have little alternative but to accept the care provided by the National Health Service (NHS). The invisibility of minority ethnic women is particularly worrying given that their own experiences are often very different from those of the mainstream: most recent arrivals will have been exposed to a traditional model of managing childbirth in which female relatives play a very influential role. These differences provide further arguments for much needed research which will contribute to our understanding of how minority ethnic women negotiate care when faced with conflicting models of childbirth. Although cultural values and traditions are constantly evolving, some values and belief systems survive despite external pressure (Bhopal 1986; Drury 1991), and the issues they raise will continue to influence the behaviour of women from these communities for the foreseeable future.

Although a small but growing body of literature has begun to address this situation by involving South Asian women in research, the subjects of this research are often treated as if they are a homogeneous group, disguising the enormous variations in experience which can be attributed to age, religious belief, socio-economic and educational background, language and patterns of migration.

People from India, Pakistan and Bangladesh are sometimes referred to as Asians or South Asians in the UK, and as East Indians in a North American context (Birbalsingh 1997). These terms often cause confusion because they are sometimes used imprecisely to describe a complex population (Bhopal *et al.* 1991). To add to this confusion, people from the Indian subcontinent are also referred to as 'coloured' and 'ethnic minority'; even though about 50 per cent of people of ethnic minority origin are born in Britain recent research sometimes also refers to them as 'immigrants' (OPCS 1991).

The presence of people of South Asian origin is not a recent phenomenon as small numbers have lived in Britain for the last few centuries (Visram 1986). However, the bulk of the South Asian population is made up of people who arrived in Britain from India and Pakistan after the Second World War, followed by a second wave of immigration from East Africa in the late seventies and later from Bangladesh (Walvin 1984; Adams 1987; Ballard 1994). Estimates from the 1991 Census suggest that 3 per cent (around 1.43 million people) of the total British population is made up of people whose roots were in the Indian subcontinent. Of these, 823,000 were Indian, 449,000 were Pakistani and 157,000 were Bangladeshi (OPCS 1991).

One of the major differences between the various South Asian communities is that they do not speak the same language. For example, in India there are more than 150 languages, none of which is spoken by more than 30 per cent of the population (Edwards 1994). In Pakistan, Urdu is the national language but other major regional languages, including Pushto, Punjabi (and Mirpuri), Baluchi and Sindhi are also spoken (Lewis 1994). In Bangladesh, dialects such as Sylheti are also spoken in addition to Bengali, the national language (Katzner 1977; Hussain 1991).

The people of the Indian subcontinent also differ in their religious beliefs. The main religions practised in the region are Hinduism, Sikhism and Islam. Islam is further divided into two main groupings, Sunnis and Shias. Within each of these two groups there are still further divisions into sects (Lewis 1994). Hindus are also divided not only into different religious sects but also into distinct caste groups (Burghart 1987; Dwyer 1994). Sikhism, likewise, is characterized by diversity.

In addition to the significant differences in patterns of migration, length of settlement and educational and occupational backgrounds, the huge disparity in economic status sets these communities apart from each other (see, for instance, Modood *et al.* 1997).

It is evident that the superficial homogeneity of people from the Indian subcontinent not only masks many important differences between the main South Asian communities in Britain, but also further differences within and between subgroups. One of the main objectives of this book is to explore some of these differences in relation to childbirth and, more pertinently, to examine the impact of traditional and medical models of childbirth practices from the perspectives of two groups of South Asian women. The women whose experiences of childbirth are the subject of this book were drawn from predominantly Hindu Gujarati Indian, and Muslim Bangladeshi communities.

## Gujarati Hindu community

Although the Gujarati Indians originate from the state of Gujarat in the north west region of India, their history of immigration is highly chequered, sometimes involving settlement in more than one continent before arriving in Britain. For example, while many Gujaratis migrated directly to Britain in the 1950s, some first settled in east and central Africa and later migrated to Britain in the late 1970s. Despite the different routes of migration and settlement patterns, many features of Gujarati culture and traditional values have survived and are strongly adhered to in Britain. For example, many Gujaratis are followers of the Hindu religion and Gujarati remains the first language for many, particularly older people. Similarly, despite the influence of British culture, their dietary habits and their mode of dress have largely remained unchanged. Other features which have been retained are the organization of the community into various caste groups and the structure and composition of the family. Although by no means universal, the extended family is still an important aspect of the Gujarati community with two or more generations of the family living under one roof. The level of literacy and educational attainment is fairly high with many men and women holding professional qualifications. The Gujaratis, particularly those from East Africa, are considered to be among the most successful South Asian immigrants to Britain (Robinson 1996; Modood *et al.* 1997).

## Bangladeshi Muslim community

The migration of the Bangladeshis from the then East Bengal or East Pakistan, and now Bangladesh, to Britain runs parallel to that of Gujaratis. The migration from East Bengal was predominantly from Sylhet – a district in the north east region of Bangladesh. The early migrants to Britain from Bangladesh were men who worked on cargo ships as sailors and cooks who later gave up their seafaring careers and settled in sea-ports around Britain (Adams 1987; Eade 1990). Unlike the Gujaratis, the migration of wives and other dependent members of the family has been a very recent phenomenon prompted by the increasing desire of many Bangladeshi men to make Britain a permanent home for themselves and their families (Carey and Shukur 1985). Because the migration of the whole family has been a relatively recent event, the Bangladeshi community has retained much closer physical and emotional links with Bangladesh, particularly as many family members have been permanently separated by the strict immigration policy introduced in the post-1970s period. The fragmentation of families across continents has had serious repercussions on the tradition of the extended family system and on informal social support networks.

All Bangladeshis are predominantly followers of Islam. Bengali is the national language but people from the Sylhet district speak the Sylheti dialect. Evidence suggests a low level of education and professional qualifications, particularly among women, and a generally low level of literacy in Bengali and English (LMP 1985; HEA 1994). The unusually high rates of unemployment and underemployment experienced by people in the Bangladeshi community make it one of the most deprived communities in Britain (House of Commons Home Affairs Committee 1986; Modood *et al.* 1997). It has also been reported that of the main South Asian communities, the Bangladeshi community has the lowest level of home ownership, with a majority renting their homes from local councils. Bangladeshi families are often housed in substandard homes lacking many basic facilities (Owen 1994; Eade *et al.* 1996).

## About the book

The main text of the book is based on in-depth interviews with 15 Gujarati and 15 Bangladeshi women in the third trimester of pregnancy and within six weeks of birth. Additional interviews were conducted with key informants from the Bangladeshi community, namely community liaison workers and maternity hospital interpreter/link workers. The interviews with the Gujarati women were carried out by the author in Gujarati. Interviews with the key informants and two of the Bangladeshi women were also conducted by the author, but in English. The remaining interviews with Bangladeshi women were carried out by bilingual interviewers who were given training in conducting in-depth interviews. Hospital obstetric notes for the Bangladeshi women were used to augment information given during face-to-face interviews.

The women were aged between 18 and 40 years and included both primipara and multiparous women. Although the individual circumstances of women in each community varied, the sample reflects the general characteristics of the communities in question. For example, the majority of Gujarati women had lived in Britain from early childhood; many had professional qualifications and were in full-time employment, owned their homes and were in a financially secure position. In marked contrast, with the exception of two women, the majority of Bangladeshi women had lived in Britain less than ten years, and lived in rented accommodation, including temporary hostels. Very few Bangladeshi women were literate in Bengali or in English and none of them had any experience of working outside their homes.

The material in the book is organized in seven chapters which trace the progress of the Gujarati and Bangladeshi women from the third trimester of pregnancy to six weeks after birth. Chapter 2 opens with a brief overview of literature on the health of South Asian women drawing on research literature on maternal and child health, access and uptake of maternity services and recent development in research on women's health issues. Chapter 3 examines women's attitudes towards conception and pregnancy and highlights the social, cultural and intergenerational differences in attitudes towards pregnancy and motherhood, and the struggles women encountered in coming to terms with pregnancy. Chapter 4 explores the women's experiences of negotiating care during pregnancy and the strategies they used to cope with the medical and traditional management of pregnancy. Chapter 5 examines differences in the women's attitudes towards, and participation in, parentcraft classes and provides an insight into their experiences of giving birth in hospital. It also discusses the extent to which knowledge of the medical procedures involved in managing labour and delivery in hospital helped or hindered the women's decisions. Chapter 6 contrasts the women's experiences of postnatal care in hospital with traditional approaches and examines the impact of the differences on the women and on other members of their families. The tension between medical and traditional models of childbirth and differences in attitudes towards pregnancy and childbirth which form central themes of the preceding chapters are developed and explored in case studies of childbirth in two Gujarati extended households. The final chapter provides an overview of the position of South Asian women in the context of British culture and current ideology surrounding childbirth practices in Britain.

## Annotated bibliography

Modood, T., Berthoud, R., Lakey, J., Nazroo, J., Smith, P., Virdee, S. and Belshon, S. (1997) *Ethnic Minorities in Britain: Diversity and Disadvantage*. London: Policy Studies Institute

This collection is based on the fourth national survey carried out by the Policy Studies Institute and it provides a comprehensive account of the experiences of ethnic minorities since the 1960s. The series of papers covers a range of key issues which have had a major impact on the experiences of ethnic minorities. Some of the most significant changes reported relate to changes in demography, family and household structure, socio-economic position, cultural identity, health, education, employment and experiences of racial harassment.

# 2

# Perspectives on South Asian mothers

## Introduction

Pregnancy and childbirth are essentially biological events, but their meanings and values are constructed and judged by the society in which these events take place. The interpretation and transmission of the values attached to these events have varied over time and across cultures. Any discussion of pregnancy and childbirth from the perspective of South Asian women needs to be examined within the framework both of their own social and cultural traditions and of those operating within the wider community of which they are also a part. The aim of this chapter is to scrutinize key research findings relating to issues concerning women's health generally and their experiences of childbirth in particular.

## Research on the health of Asians in Britain

The main focus of research on the health of South Asians in Britain was, for a long time, on specific or so-called 'exotic' diseases associated with 'immigrants'. Initially, diseases such as tuberculosis (Clarke *et al.* 1979), rickets (Swan and Cooke 1971; Goel *et al.* 1981), mental disorder (Littlewood and Lipsedge 1982) and certain inherited conditions were singled out for investigation.

Critics argue that researchers in the past have relied on simplistic interpretations based on cultural differences and individual behaviour rather than on the socio-economic circumstances of people to explain the cause of poor health (Ahmad *et al.* 1989; Sheldon and Parker 1992; Ahmad 1993). For example, the prevalence of particular illnesses or diseases was attributed to cultural practices such as dietary habits, marriage patterns or individual behaviour, ignoring the fact that factors which determine health status are more complex.

The lack of consideration given to theoretical and methodological issues in health research on ethnic minorities is equally striking for a number of reasons. This particularly applies in relation to the use of the term 'race' or ethnicity. Not only are these concepts poorly defined but are often used imprecisely and inappropriately to explain differences in health outcomes. Although race is essentially a social construct which reflects social structures and relationships based on power, it is often used as a category to explain differences in health outcomes. In the same vein, ethnicity is often narrowly defined in terms of culture whereas ethnicity is a complex entity which encompasses not only aspects of physical appearance but ideas of national identity, shared cultural traditions such as diet, dress and language, and religious traditions (Smaje 1995). The simplistic interpretations of ethnicity in research have not only encouraged cultural stereotypes but also various broadly defined cultural groups have been treated as if they were homogeneous, with static values and belief systems. In the process, enormous differences between and within South Asian communities, not only in terms of culture, language and religion but also with respect to socio-economic and migration histories, have largely been overlooked.

Further, critics argue that bias in research is also apparent from the fact that much of the previous health research on ethnic minorities was carried out to further the interests of health professionals rather than those of the communities being researched (Bhopal 1992; Sheldon and Parker 1992). Although a growing body of literature is emerging which is beginning to involve minority ethnic groups in setting the agenda for research and in examining health concerns from the perspective of the communities concerned, this is a relatively recent phenomenon.

## South Asian women's experiences of health

Following the first wave of research into rickets and infectious diseases, attention shifted to black and Asian women's experiences of pregnancy, birth and maternity care. Initially, the main focus was on birth statistics, perinatal mortality, low birthweight and congenital malformations. The research in this area was characterized by a lack of consistency in approach and a failure to justify the singling out of minority ethnic women in this way while excluding them from the studies exploring the concerns of the women in general.

Phoenix (1990a) and Parsons *et al.* (1993), among others, point out that by limiting the field of enquiry to a small number of problematic areas, researchers have created the impression that minority ethnic women are generally more predisposed to obstetric 'risk' than their white counterparts. For example, higher rates of perinatal mortality, low birthweight and congenital malformations have become synonymous with black and Asian babies. Until recently, it was generally assumed that mortality rates in babies born to minority ethnic women were similarly high across all groups.

Evidence from in-depth analyses of birth statistics for England and Wales (Balarajan and Botting 1989; Balarajan and Raleigh 1990) reveals a complex pattern of stillbirths and infant mortality rates across England and Wales, with a marked variation in the patterns of stillbirths, neonatal and postnatal mortality in babies born to women from India, Pakistan and Bangladesh.

Congenital malformations have been identified as one of the major causes of infant deaths among babies born to Pakistani mothers (Gillies *et al.* 1984; Chitty and Winter 1989). However, despite the large volume of research in this area, the evidence is inconclusive and contentious. For example, findings of some studies have linked high rates of infant mortality to congenital malformations and consanguineous (mainly first cousin) marriages (Bundey *et al.* 1989; Chitty and Winter 1989). Yet, the findings of other studies suggest that marriages between first cousins provide only a partial explanation for the unusually high rates of infant deaths (see, for example, Honeyman *et al.* 1987; Pearson 1991). In fact, Ahmad (1996b: 68), in his critical analysis of the literature on congenital abnormality and consanguinity, asserts that consanguinity simply offers a convenient explanation whereas in reality it is far more difficult to isolate the relative contribution of potentially explanatory factors, such as genetic inheritance, age of mother, parity, environmental causes and access to and quality of medical care.

The low birthweight of babies born to mothers in some minority ethnic communities has also been a popular area of research because it was assumed that full term babies weighing less than five pounds were at an increased risk of perinatal morbidity and mortality. The fact that the birthweights of Asian babies were measured against the standard growth charts and tables constructed for British indigenous babies was not considered to be problematic. This is a highly questionable practice since these charts do not take into account the genetic make-up of parents or the stature of their mothers. Evidence from studies on birthweight of babies in America casts further doubt on the association between low birthweight and perinatal mortality (Institute of Medicine 1985, cited in Phoenix 1990a).

Although the association between low birthweight and perinatal mortality remains tentative, 'inappropriate' and 'inadequate' diet is often cited as the main reason for the low birthweights of babies born to Asian mothers. This preoccupation with the Asian diet has prompted various attempts (Bissenden 1979; Wharton 1982; Haines *et al.* 1982) to establish the link between low birthweight and Asian women's diet during pregnancy. Despite numerous studies on Asian diets and low birthweight, the evidence remains inconclusive, especially when pregnant women of social classes I and II were studied (Rush 1982; Abraham *et al.* 1985). It is unfortunate that the narrow focus on dietary habits detracts attention from important causes such as social and material deprivation (Runnymede Trust and Radical Statistics Group 1980).

## Experiences of maternity care

Generally women of childbearing age and those with small children are more likely than any other group to have an increased need of health care services. Since the beginning of this century, the state and the medical profession have had a major impact on childbirth practices in Britain because of the growing concern with infant mortality and later with maternal health. Fertility, pregnancy and childbirth have increasingly become seen as medical events. However, it is important to stress that this trend has also been noted in many other aspects of human life. For example, Illich (1976) and Zola (1978) provide interesting insights into how medicine has assumed control over decisions affecting various aspects of human life such as death, pain, public health, pollution, lifestyles and environmental health.

Although there is considerable controversy about the factors contributing to poor birth outcome, cultural practices and beliefs about pregnancy and childbirth have often been blamed for the poor uptake of maternity services. It has been widely reported that South Asian women generally have a poor record of attendance at antenatal clinics, and in some cases women do not present themselves at the clinic until very late in their pregnancies (Clarke and Clayton 1983; Jain 1985; Clarke and Clayton *et al.* 1988; Firdous and Bhopal 1989; Parsons *et al.* 1993). The solution seems to lie in more regular attendance at clinics and better advice about diet in pregnancy.

The Asian Mother and Baby Campaign, an initiative funded by the Department of Health, was launched in 1984 specifically to improve obstetric outcome for South Asian women. The campaign had two main features: first, a programme of publicity and health education to raise awareness about the importance of antenatal care in the South Asian community and second, the provision of link-workers to bridge the language barrier between Asian mothers and health professionals and at the same time encourage local health authorities to develop services which were sensitive to the needs of South Asian women (Rocheron 1988).

The campaign was received with a great deal of scepticism because it was modelled on the much-criticized 'Stop Rickets' campaign and had inherited many of its ideological and methodological weaknesses. The campaign's goals and agenda were set by health professionals and reflected their priorities while the issues affecting the women in question were not taken into consideration. The campaign messages placed undue emphasis on cultural values and poor dietary habits while paying scant regard to the complexity and diversity of the South Asian population including correlation between infant mortality and the mothers' social and material circumstances. For example, there is direct evidence linking high rates of infant mortality to social and economic deprivation among families with fathers in manual occupations, a group which includes a significant proportion of the minority ethnic population (Townsend and Davidson 1982; Pharoah and Alberman 1990; Whitehead 1992). It was also significant that, although some of the major barriers to maternity services are rooted in individual and institutionalized racism, the campaign largely failed to address the question of racism within maternity services (for a critique of these initiatives see, for instance, Donovan 1983; Rocheron 1988).

While clinical antenatal care has a useful role in the early detection and prevention of certain conditions, treating all South Asian women as being potentially at equal risk is to deny the immense diversity in the utilization of maternity services by different groups of South Asian women (see, for instance, Dobson 1988 and Woollett *et al.* 1995). Furthermore, a number of researchers (Enkin and Chalmers 1982; Enkin *et al.* 1990; Tew 1990; Steer 1993 among others) have cast considerable doubt on the effectiveness of clinical antenatal care. One of the main criticisms of the present form of routine antenatal care is that while it subjects all women to a range of screening tests, it is not effective in predicting and detecting preventable problems:

> It is true that the screening tests are by and large non-invasive and free from direct hazard, but this in no way implies that there is no risk associated with their use. Their potential for harm derives primarily from their capacity for erroneously indicating the presence of pathology. The suspicion thus engendered may lead to heightened anxiety, or more seriously, to unwarranted intervention for the 'prevention' or 'treatment' of non-disease.
>
> (Enkin and Chalmers 1982: 270)

It is also important to recognize that uptake of antenatal services depends on the quality of care provided and the extent to which women feel their needs are met (Parsons and Day 1992). The quality of services provided and the attitudes of mothers towards antenatal care clearly need to be seen within the broader context of environmental and social factors and institutional structures. A number of mitigating factors affect access to, and the quality of maternity care services provided by, general practitioners. Although there is diversity within the South Asian population, a majority live in the more deprived parts of the inner city with traditionally higher morbidity and mortality rates than in the more affluent areas, and with primary health care services overstretched and unable to cope with the level of demand (MORI 1993; Smaje 1995). Consequently, the quality of maternity care that is available is outside the control of women who have the greatest need. Clarke and Clayton's (1983) findings, for example, revealed that the standard of antenatal care provided by general practitioners was highly variable; general practitioners of South Asian women offered poor quality of care on a number of indicators of quality. Other researchers have expressed similar concerns about poor access to, and quality of, care provided to South Asian women (Stonham and Sims 1986; Lone 1987).

Apart from poor access to maternity services, various studies (Garcia 1982; Jackson-Baker 1988; Gladman 1994) have concluded that, for women generally, the experience of antenatal care is less than satisfactory. As well as sharing some of the common problems with other women, such as having to make a long journey to keep hospital appointments, transportation costs, responsibility for other children and long waiting times at the clinic, it has been suggested that many women from the minority ethnic communities are prevented from making effective use of the maternity services due to language and communication problems, intrusive examinations, the lack of explanations, negative stereotyping and the racist attitudes of health professionals (Phoenix 1990a; Bowler 1993). Bowler's (1993) exploration of nurses and midwives' interactions with South Asian mothers exposes the extent to which negative stereotyping and racist attitudes determine the quality of care provided. Some of the common stereotypes of Asian women were found to be an inability to speak English, a lack of compliance with care, abuse or overuse of the service, a tendency to 'make a fuss about nothing' and a lack of maternal instinct (Bowler 1993: 160).

Examples of negative perceptions of women from minority ethnic groups are also evident in the midwifery and nursing literature. Much of the literature is confined to describing cultural practices relating to pregnancy and childbirth. Beard (1982), for instance, compares the use of contraception by a group of women in minority ethnic communities with a small control group of unmatched white women. The examination of the family planning practices of the Asian women in the context of cultural and religious beliefs serves only to highlight the stereotypical images of arranged marriages and large numbers of children. Very often Bangladeshi women are used as an example of women with high parity, though there has been little or no exploration of the women's views about fertility and family planning. Instead it is assumed that, with time and the guidance of the health professionals, the attitude of the next generation of Asian women will be brought into line with those of the indigenous women:

> It is clear that members of the ethnic groups studied are retaining many of their cultural ideals, which are often in conflict with limiting family size. This is in spite of all the free family planning services that are available. It will take several generations to alter ingrained modes of life but it is up to us health educators to provide knowledge about contraception in order to prevent further overcrowding, ill health and hardship in families already overburdened with problems.
>
> (Beard 1982: 421)

Charles's (1983) and Phillips's (1985) studies also make gross generalizations about Asian cultures and religion based on superficial observations. Implicit in the generalizations is the expectation that if only all Asian women could be encouraged to abandon their cultural habits in favour of 'western' dress and, in particular, 'western' diet, their problems would disappear. For instance, Charles (1983) considers the Asian diet to be nutritionally unsound and sees the adoption of the English diet as a desirable outcome for women conforming to the western 'ideal': 'Many Asians are now inclined to eat English food but even if they eat chapattis they will eat meat as they now seem to realise that their diet is not very nutritious.'

Such studies are frequently disseminated in nursing journals and magazines in order that researchers might share their knowledge and experience with other health workers, thus serving to perpetuate stereotypes without exploring the real concerns of the Asian women in question. When the views of health providers have been coloured by negative images and misconceptions, this has serious implications for the provision of unbiased care and medical advice.

While there is no shortage of literature focusing on the medical problems of Asian women from the perspective of the medical and nursing professions, as we shall see, there have been only a small number of studies which have explored childbirth from the perspectives of South Asian mothers. Sometimes this has had unfortunate effects. For example, Donovan (1984) and Pearson (1983, 1986), among others, have pointed out that the definition of research questions by the majority group is likely to create a series of difficulties. These include both the identification of the whole range of health issues affecting minority ethnic communities, and the accessibility and uptake of the health services:

> Those who have 'integrated' (i.e. assimilated/become British) are clearly not a problem; it is those who steadfastly refuse to do so. Muslim women who are seen as 'cloistered' or 'imprisoned' in purdah cause 'problems' for services such as the National Health Service when they attend clinics and neither speak English nor submit to the requirements that they should be examined by a male doctor . . . The responsibility for communication and 'integration' lies (un)fairly and squarely at the door of the minority that speaks an 'alien' language.
>
> (Pearson 1983: 38)

## Development in research on women's health issues

This bias in research is in marked contrast to developments within the maternity services which have responded to the needs of women in the white community. Such developments are the result of a great deal of research which has specifically addressed the issues surrounding childbirth from women's point of view (see, for instance, Kitzinger 1962; Oakley 1979, 1980; Graham and McKee 1980; MacIntyre 1981; McIntosh 1989). By focusing on childbirth from the women's perspective, writers such as Ann Oakley and Sheila Kitzinger have highlighted the concerns many women have about current childbirth practices.

The recent trend towards hospital delivery for all women with the increased risk of medical intervention has become a major concern for many women because it effectively deprives them of the opportunity of exercising any control during childbirth. It is generally accepted that a small number of women are 'at risk' and may require constant medical supervision throughout their pregnancy and childbirth. It has, however, been strongly argued that it is not necessary for all women to give birth in hospital or to be subjected to unnecessary medical intervention (Kitzinger and Davis 1978; Oakley 1984).

While the debate about whether women or professionals should control childbirth continues (see, for instance, Oakley 1984; Campbell and Macfarlane 1990), research which examines women's experiences of childbirth has helped to challenge the attitudes of the medical profession towards a number of medical procedures. Some studies have investigated specific aspects of medical intervention during pregnancy and childbirth. For example, women's experiences of epidurals (Kitzinger 1987) and episiotomy (Kitzinger and Walter 1981) have helped to highlight the implications of these procedures for women who did not require them or were not helped by them. Other modern childbirth practices which have attracted a great deal of interest are the number of unnecessary inductions and Caesarean deliveries (Cartwright 1979; Oakley 1984; Oakley and Richards 1990).

While there is no shortage of literature on childbirth which specifically addresses issues from white women's point of view, the notion of Asian women as consumers has rarely been addressed. It is unfortunate that so few researchers in the field of childbirth have included black and minority ethnic women in their investigations, using shortage of funding and language barriers to justify the exclusion of non-English speaking women from their studies. In many national surveys of women's experiences of childbirth (Green *et al.* 1990; Green 1993), with the exception of the survey on infant feeding practices (Thomas and Avery 1997), there is very little indication that black and Asian women were included in the surveys and, if the sample did include non-white women, how their experiences compared with the white women.

Although there is a particular dearth of literature on childbirth from the perspective of South Asian women, a small but growing volume of literature is emerging to remedy the situation. A number of recent studies have evaluated the quality of care provided to South Asian women in pregnancy and in the postnatal period. For example, Narang and Murphy (1994) carried out interviews with a small group of Asian mothers in the antenatal period to assess their knowledge and understanding about tests and screening procedures. Their findings suggested that half of the women did not know the nature of the tests performed on them and only a handful of them knew the reasons why these tests were performed. They concluded that women who lacked information and explanations about different screening procedures were denied opportunities to make informed decisions about their care and to play an active role in the management of pregnancy.

Theodore-Gandi and Shaikh (1988) carried out interviews with 74 Asian and 74 white women to compare their experiences of maternity care. They concluded that the Asian women were less likely than white women to be offered any choice in pain relief or delivery position. In similar vein, evidence from a recent pilot evaluation about the acceptability and usefulness of leaflets on *Positions in Labour and Routine Ultrasound* (NHS/CRD 1996) revealed that women who did not speak English were less likely to be given information leaflets about positions in labour or ultrasound by midwifery staff. It would appear that many midwifery staff made an arbitrary judgement about which group of pregnant women should have a right to receive information leaflets. It is perhaps not very surprising that the level of knowledge about the nature and range of medical procedures involved in the management of labour and delivery, including information about pain relief and positions in labour, among South Asian women is generally very low (Firdous and Bhopal 1989).

Apart from the small amount of literature on Asian women's views on maternity care, a number of qualitative studies have examined the experiences of pregnancy and childbirth from the perspectives of South Asian women (Homans 1980; Dobson 1988; Woollett and Dosanjh-Matwala 1990a; Woollett *et al.* 1995). Homans (1980), for example, follows the progress of Asian and white women through their pregnancies to compare their perceptions of maternal health services, the resources they used and the nature and extent of support given by social networks. The Asian women were of Punjabi origin but belonged to different religious groups; about half were Sikh and the rest were Muslim and Hindus. Her findings suggest that there were many similarities and differences between Asian and white women's experiences of pregnancy. The similarities between Asian and white women were evident at several levels, for instance with respect to the status of women in society, their role as mothers, and the use of traditional remedies in the management of minor ailments in pregnancy, including shared notions of prescriptions and restrictions for maintaining health in pregnancy. Examples of prescriptions and restrictions included the beliefs about pollution surrounding menstruation and childbirth and observance of rites and rituals to safeguard the health of mother and her unborn child and, additionally for Asian women, modification of diet based on the beliefs in 'hot' and 'cold' properties of foods. As we shall see later in Chapter 4, similar beliefs about prescriptions and proscriptions are important aspects of managing the care of pregnant women in many other cultures across the world (Pillsbury 1978; Messer 1981; Lozoff *et al.* 1988).

Homans's findings (1980) also suggested that the differences between Asian and white women were reflected mainly in cultural and religious beliefs; for example, Asian women's views about the 'ideal' number of children were more likely to be influenced by their religious beliefs as were their views about taboos associated with menstruation and childbirth. In addition, the differences in the organization of the family, such as the tradition of the extended family structure and the influential role of mothers-in-law in supervising the proscriptions and prescriptions relating to diet and behaviour during pregnancy and in overseeing the observance of rituals to comply with pollution taboos, were more commonly reported by Asian women than by white women. Homans argues that differences in socio-economic position, parity and educational attainment were equally important in shaping the women's experiences of negotiating maternity care and in their ability to comply with medical advice.

In another study, Dobson (1988) carried out retrospective interviews with a small group of Sikh and Muslim Punjabi mothers who had at least one child under five years old. Dobson draws broadly similar conclusions about the influence of culture and religion, the role of female relatives and the rules governing prescriptions and restrictions during pregnancy and after childbirth. She discusses the importance Sikh and Muslim mothers attached to their beliefs in the omnipotent god while at the same time believing in the power of evil forces or spirits who could do harm to the pregnant mother and her unborn child. The maintenance of dietary habits according to 'hot' and 'cold' foods principles and the role of rituals were regarded as important elements of traditional childbirth practices. However, Dobson reiterates the point made by Homans that although the experiences of Asian women were influenced by traditional childbirth practices, this did not make the medically orientated childbirth practices less acceptable to them.

Woollett and associates (1995) use a similar line of enquiry to that of Homans by comparing the experiences of pregnancy and childbirth of Asian women and white women in East London. Their study includes Asian women from Hindu, Muslim and Sikh communities who were either fluent in English or were fluent in Hindi, Urdu and Punjabi but excludes Asian women from other linguistic groups. Evidence from their study suggests that, while cultural and religious beliefs had a strong influence on Asian women's perceptions of pregnancy and childbirth, the degree of familiarity with the western childbirth practices, including fluency in English, had a significant impact on Asian women's perceptions of their pregnancy and childbirth. They argue that Asian women who had lived in the UK for a long time were more likely to be fluent in English, and consequently more likely to be knowledgeable about maternity care and to want their husbands to be present at the time of delivery. Their findings, however, do not support the evidence concerning the level of practical help and advice offered by female relatives to pregnant women reported by other studies. For example, they report that the level of support provided by female relatives was less than that reported by Homans and Dobson, and that many mothers in nuclear families were more likely to be supported by their husbands and friends than members of their extended family. They also assert that Asian women's ideas and experiences of pregnancy and childbirth need to be seen in a broader context and not merely in relation to women's ethnicity and religion.

While these studies have made a valuable contribution by opening up discussion, a wide gap in knowledge about the views of South Asian women on a range of medical interventions, such as the use of pain relief, Caesarean sections, induction and episiotomy, still remains. For example, there is evidence to suggest that instrumental delivery involving the use of forceps, vacuum extractors and Caesarean section is particularly high among some women in the ethnic minority groups (Parsons *et al.* 1993) and yet we know relatively little about the views of black and Asian women concerning the impact of some of these procedures on their lives.

## Summary

To sum up then, a review of literature reveals a number of unmistakable trends. In various different fields, including education and anthropology, the tendency has been for the majority group to define the 'problem' and, very often, to locate the cause of the problem firmly in the minority communities themselves. In a similar vein, researchers have very often grouped together ethnic minorities as a homogeneous, monolithic whole, failing to perceive the tremendous social and cultural diversity which marks the many different groups. This tendency is certainly a recurrent feature of research on health: all too often medical researchers not only define the problems without consultation with the communities concerned but, explicitly or implicitly, suggest that the causes of these problems are located within the communities themselves. The research reported in the chapters which follow is an attempt to avoid these pitfalls, and approaches the question of women's experiences of pregnancy and childbirth from the perspectives of two different groups of Asian women. The women were drawn from the Bangladeshi Muslim and Gujarati Hindu communities. The women in these two communities were chosen because of the differences in their cultural, social and migration histories and socio-economic positions within British society. It is also evident from the previous research on Asian women's experiences of childbirth that for many Asian women traditional and medical models of managing care during pregnancy and childbirth were very much part and parcel of their lives. The book also attempts to develop this theme further by examining strategies Gujarati and Bangladeshi women use to negotiate between medical and traditional models of care.

## Annotated bibliography

Ahmad, W.I.U. (ed.) (1993) *'Race' and Health in Contemporary Britain*. Buckingham: Open University Press.
This collection of papers provides an analysis of the health and health care of Britain's black population within the context of political, economic and institutional structures and the ideology of racism. In this series, the essay by Parsons and colleagues provides a critical analysis of research literature on maternity care for black and ethnic minority women. The main focus of review is on the methods of data collection and on the interpretation of the results. The authors draw attention to the poor quality of data which has informed much of the previous research on perinatal mortality and the maternal health of ethnic minority women and discuss its implications for policy and practice.

Phoenix, A. (1990) 'Black women and the maternity services', in J. Garcia, R. Kilpatrick and M. Richards (eds) *The Politics of Maternity Care: Services for Childbearing Women in Twentieth-Century Britain*. Oxford: Clarendon.
This paper explores the relationship between ethnic minority women and the maternity services. The discussion considers the ways in which racial discrimination is institutionalized in the maternity services and the problems it creates for black and Asian women in accessing maternity care. It also assesses some of the initiatives that have been set up to address the needs of black and Asian women.
Rocheron, Y. (1988) The Asian Mother and Baby Campaign: the construction of ethnic minorities' health needs, *Critical Social Policy*, 22: 4–23.
This paper is based on an external evaluation of the Asian Mother and Baby Campaign and provides critical analysis of the effectiveness of the campaign, highlighting the reasons for the lack of effectiveness in meeting the maternity care needs of South Asian mothers.

# 3

# Experiences of becoming pregnant

Pregnancy, childbirth and motherhood are important biological facts in the life cycle of women. However, they are also social and cultural experiences. The meaning and values attached to them are defined and shaped by prevalent social norms and cultural traditions (Wolkind and Zajicek 1981; MacCormack 1982; Phoenix *et al.* 1991). It has been suggested by Richardson (1993) and Oakley (1980), for instance, that popular ideas about pregnancy and childbirth are based on cultural stereotypes about feminine characteristics. They argue that the cultural stereotypes about women and their childbearing role are unhelpful because they fail to acknowledge that women are more than just the sum total of their biology and these events do not take place in a social vacuum. This bias in the construction and interpretation of pregnancy, childbirth and motherhood is not restricted to the more popular views but is also evident in anthropological, psychological, sociological and medical literature.

The writings of Homans (1980), MacCormack (1982) and Currer (1986), among others, provide interesting examples of culture-specific differences in attitudes towards pregnancy and motherhood. Evidence suggests that, irrespective of culture, the social position and the role of women in biological reproduction are governed by the collective ideologies of the social institutions. Analyses of feminist literature point, in particular, to the roles of the state, religion, law and medicine in defining ideas about women and their role in biological reproduction (Oakley 1984; Homans 1985a; Phoenix *et al.* 1991). Similarly, attitudes towards the status of Asian women and their childbearing role are reflected in the ideology of patriarchy, caste, class and religion systems (Hussain and Radwan 1984; Liddle and Joshi 1986; Jeffery *et al.* 1989).

Homans (1985a), Phoenix (1990b) and Richardson (1993) have argued that explanations for society's attitudes towards pregnancy and motherhood can only be understood within the context of the sexual politics of reproduction. Its impact is most evident in relation to the social control of female sexuality, fertility and family planning and in the medical management of pregnancy and childbirth. For example, social attitudes towards female sexuality and fertility not only determine which group of women should or should not be encouraged to become pregnant but also the circumstances in which they should do so. Social control over fertility determines that only a pregnancy occurring within the context of marriage is approved, although there has been some shift in attitude in this regard.

Although unmarried mothers in Britain no longer suffer the same degree of ostracism, traditional views on marriage and motherhood still prevail. While there is a degree of tolerance towards unmarried mothers within the white community, there is a less tolerant attitude in South Asian communities and this acts as a repressive mechanism for controlling female fertility (Day 1994). For instance, the position of unmarried mothers within the South Asian communities is unenviable because sexual relationships outside marriage are regarded as immoral acts. Since the shame and dishonour attached to such liaisons affect all members of the family, extra care is taken to guard female sexuality and fertility. Such attitudes towards control over female fertility not only exist in the Indian subcontinent (cf. Caplan 1985; Aziz and Maloney 1985; Jeffery *et al.* 1989) but also continue to influence the attitude and behaviour of people within the British South Asian communities.

Oakley (1980) and Graham (1977), among others, point to the large volume of research on childbirth experiences of married women which suggests that, until recently, researchers were equally guilty of adhering to prevailing 'social norms' by confining their interest exclusively to married women having their first baby. Consequently, pregnant women who were already mothers or those who were unmarried were rarely invited to give their views about their experiences of pregnancy. While this bias has largely been corrected by studies which have included multiparous women and single and teenage mothers in the white community (Cunningham 1984; Phoenix 1990b), there is still a dearth of literature on black and Asian women's views of conception and motherhood.

The paucity of literature on this subject is particularly striking given that black and Asian women's fertility behaviour has received a great deal of interest from health professionals and researchers alike. This is evident from the large volume of studies which have focused primarily on family planning practices among Asian women (Zaklama 1984; McAvoy and Raza 1988; Day 1994). This emphasis has been matched by the vast quantity of health education literature on birth control targeted specifically at Asian women (Phoenix 1990a; Bhopal and White 1993). It has been argued that this focus is based on the racist assumption that Asian women have far too many babies (Bowler 1993).

Although the studies by Homans (1980), Dobson (1988) and Woollett and Dosanjh-Matwala (1990a) provide some useful information about Asian women's experiences of their pregnancies, their analyses do not include information about women's attitudes to conception and pregnancy or the extent to which these were coloured by their personal and social circumstances. In this chapter I wish to focus on two separate issues in an attempt to redress this imbalance: first, I will explore attitudes of Gujarati and Bangladeshi women towards conception and motherhood; and second, I will examine the women's initial reactions to their pregnancies. As we shall see later, these issues had major implications for the way they managed their pregnancies and childbirth.

## Asian women's attitudes to conception and motherhood

Evidence from the literature on the white community suggests that a woman's personal and social circumstances can have a major influence on her attitude towards her pregnancy and her as yet unborn child. For example, the findings of Oakley (1979) and Wolkind and Zajicek (1981) suggest that factors such as women's own expectations of their pregnancies and motherhood, their ideas about society's expectations of their social role, their marital status, and their relationships with their husbands and other members of the family were important in determining their attitudes towards their pregnancies.

Most women have a strong biological and emotional need to bear children. The desire to bear children is also reinforced by cultural and social conditioning which affects all women irrespective of ethnic, social, cultural or religious backgrounds. Within the South Asian communities, additional factors associated with cultural and religious traditions also have a major effect on women's reproductive behaviour. For example, there is a strong obligation for women to produce children to ensure the continuity of the family line. The stigma attached to either unmarried or barren women acts as a strong discouragement for women to question the status attached to marriage and motherhood (Homans 1982; Kabeer 1985; Schott and Henley 1996).

In many respects Gujarati and Bangladeshi women's perceptions of conception and pregnancy were similar to those reported in the literature for white women (Oakley 1979; Homans 1980). For example, many women explained that although they had not given any serious thought to having children, they were aware that rejection of marriage or motherhood was unthinkable as they were expected to conform to the expected role for women: '. . . deep down I always knew that I would have to get married one day and have children. I don't think there is any choice to do otherwise. No one expects you to remain unmarried. Once you are married it is expected that you will have children' (Gujarati mother, second pregnancy).

There was also consensus among both groups of women that children were a consequence of marriage, and conception was only approved within the framework of a marriage: 'No, I never thought about it. I always believed that marriage will come first and then whatever things happen will happen anyway. Pregnancy is common and something natural' (Bangladeshi mother, seventh pregnancy).

The women's perceptions of the desirability of conception are also shaped by the subtle pressure exerted on them after marriage to have children. This often takes the form of blessings given to the married couple after marriage: 'May god bless you with many sons.' This sort of subtle pressure continues until a woman becomes pregnant. A number of Gujarati women who were expecting their first babies reported that they had been under considerable pressure to have a baby after the first year of marriage. In most cases, the pressure came from mothers-in-law or other members of the husband's family: 'My mother-in-law told my husband that we had been married over three years and yet there was no sign of a baby. She felt we had waited too long and she was beginning to suspect that there was something wrong with us' (Gujarati mother, first pregnancy).

In cultures based on a patrilineal system and an agrarian economy, having children, particularly sons, is important in order to carry forward the name of the family into future generations and also to ensure security in old age. Homans (1982), Dobson (1988) and Woollett and Donsanjh-Matwala (1990a) report that not only is a woman required to prove her fertility, but she is also expected to bear at least one son. Religious beliefs also exert similar pressures on women to produce a male child. For example, among the Gujarati Hindus, there is additional pressure on women to give birth to a male child. It is believed that unless a son performs the rituals of death, the departed person's soul does not reach heaven (Ahmed and Watt 1986). However, attitudes may vary between people.

The accounts given by a number of Bangladeshi and Gujarati women suggested that having a male child was vitally important but not all explained the importance of a male child in religious terms. It was also evident that the women's concerns about the sex of the baby reflected the interest and expectations that other people had in their pregnancy:

> Lots of people expect you to want only sons but I think the sex of the baby doesn't matter. My mother-in-law's reference to my baby is only in terms of a boy and not a girl. Overall, in my experience, there is a general expectation that I am carrying a male child!
>
> (Gujarati mother, first pregnancy)

Some first-time mothers had adopted a carefree attitude towards the sex of their baby because they were secure in the knowledge that there was still hope that their next pregnancy may produce a son. However, this optimism was not shared by all first-time mothers or by those who already had daughters but no sons. These women were less dismissive about the importance of having a son because they were aware that it would be interpreted as a sign of inadequacy and could lead to a loss of status within their family:

> I feel that there is indirect pressure on me to have a son. My mother-in-law and her friends keep reminding me that I must be carrying a boy, almost wishing it on me to have a boy. My husband's sister who is expecting her third baby recently had an amniocentesis and if the test

> had showed that it was a girl then she would have had an abortion. Fortunately for her, it is going to be a boy.
>
> (Gujarati mother, first pregnancy)

Although religious beliefs did not appear to affect Bangladeshi women's attitudes towards the sex of the baby, women who only had daughters were aware that not having a son would have far-reaching consequences for the inheritance of property:

> When my second daughter was born a few members of my family, from both sides, openly expressed their disappointment that I had failed to produce a son. They hinted that unless I produced a son, they would have to arrange the marriage of my two daughters with their cousins to ensure that my husband's inheritance remained within the family. I am aware of the kinds of comments that will be made if this baby is also a girl.
>
> (Bangladeshi mother, third pregnancy)

Consequently mothers who were desperate to have a son were prepared to go to extraordinary lengths in order to conceive a male child. Some women had followed a special diet:

> This diet recommends you to eat acidic fruits and cut down on all dairy produce. I was on this diet a few weeks after my pregnancy was confirmed. We might have a third baby if this baby is a girl. I would like to have a boy this time as most of our Indians like boys, especially fathers.
>
> (Gujarati mother, second pregnancy)

The stigma attached to the lack of a son had compelled another mother to ignore the advice of her doctor against a further pregnancy, which could have caused long-term damage to her health:

> After my second Caesarean section, the consultant at the hospital had warned me that my womb was not strong enough to withstand any more pregnancies. My doctor had also reminded me that a third pregnancy would be hazardous. I was prepared to delay it a little but had not given up the idea. I was hell bent on having a son. I was not concerned as I am now that my womb might rupture.
>
> (Bangladeshi mother, third pregnancy)

Many South Asian Muslims also believe that children are blessings from God and therefore each pregnancy should be accepted as a gift (Abdullah and Zeidenstein 1982; Ahmed 1990; Zaida 1994). It has been reported that Islamic law does not directly set out its opposition to birth control (El-Islam *et al.* 1988). Atkin *et al.* (1998) show that attitudes to termination vary between Muslim women and among the same women during different pregnancies. However, some Muslims believe that it is a sin to prevent a pregnancy and therefore would not be willing to use any form of birth control: 'We were not taking any precautions to prevent a pregnancy since the birth of my second baby. We don't go in for family planning because we think of children as blessings from God' (Bangladeshi mother, third pregnancy).

While the impact of these beliefs on women's attitudes towards conception and pregnancy may vary enormously, women's personal experiences or awareness about the worryingly high rates of infant mortality in the Indian subcontinent may also influence their behaviour. For example, Kabeer (1985) argues that although high fertility is known to be potentially detrimental to women's health, the traditional value placed on women's fertility and the fear of high infant deaths provide a powerful argument against limiting family size.

It has also been argued by Woollett *et al.* (1991) that beliefs about conception and pregnancy are modified by the process of acculturation. Their findings suggest that, irrespective of religious beliefs, factors such as the length of settlement in Britain and fluency in English were important in making women more predisposed towards family planning. Furthermore, although acculturation could account for the women's attitudes towards conception, it was evident that the women were having to strike a delicate balance between the need to fulfil religious and cultural expectations and the need for spacing and limiting the size of the family. The dilemma many women faced in negotiating the competing demands of social and cultural expectations and family planning is explored.

## Planned or unplanned pregnancy?

A planned pregnancy suggests that it was a deliberate and conscious decision to have a baby by giving up the use of contraceptives. In contrast, an unplanned pregnancy implies that the pregnancy was an accident due to the failure of contraception. However, such broad categories can mask what is actually taking place. As we will see, for some women the notion of planning a pregnancy was an alien concept since they believed that even without contraception pregnancy would not occur immediately. In a similar vein, the distinction between the 'planners' and 'non-planners' suggests that the differences are closely aligned with women's attitudes towards conception, whereas in reality there are many similarities in the attitudes of planners and non-planners.

Although the Gujarati and Bangladeshi women also fell into the two broad categories of the planned and unplanned pregnancy, the circumstances under which some of the women had found themselves pregnant were more complex and ambiguous than seemed at first. Examination of the types of contraceptive methods used and attitudes to family planning provided clues to the individual circumstances under which women had become pregnant. Just over half of Gujarati and Bangladeshi women interviewed indicated that they had stopped using contraceptives to have a baby:

> We were trying for another baby because I had lost a baby. I had a miscarriage at three months because I had carried on taking the contraceptive pill after I had become pregnant. This time my husband used condoms until it was safe for us to try again.
>
> (Bangladeshi mother, fifth pregnancy)

Apart from the women who had deliberately stopped taking precautions to have a baby, a number of women, who had never practised any form of birth control, also claimed that their pregnancy was planned because they were waiting for it just to happen: 'I did not use birth control before I became pregnant. This is my first pregnancy. I expected to become pregnant one day. We didn't try for it' (Bangladeshi mother, first pregnancy).

When the circumstances of the remaining Gujarati and Bangladeshi women, who did not wish to become pregnant, were analysed, they fell into four categories. These were: failure of contraception; a half-hearted attempt at birth control with only one partner keen on pregnancy; neither partner keen on pregnancy nor on birth control; and finally, women who accepted pregnancy as ordained by the will of God.

While the attitudes and behaviour of the women who had intended to become pregnant were self-evident, the attitudes of the women who had not consciously set out to become pregnant need further explanation. In a small number of cases, pregnancy had occurred accidentally due to contraceptive failure. In all these cases the couples were relying on the condom to prevent a pregnancy. Many women felt that they were unable to prevent their pregnancies because they depended on their husbands' attitudes to birth control and their willingness to take the responsibility for preventing pregnancy seriously: 'As I suffer from very high blood pressure I can't take any birth control pills. My husband has to use the condom. The whole pregnancy was an accident. Don't know how it happened . . . maybe it is God's will' (Bangladeshi mother, third pregnancy).

It was also evident that differences in attitudes towards birth control sometimes determined the circumstances under which some women had become pregnant. A Gujarati mother whose husband believed that the decision about birth control should be left to the man accidentally became pregnant when she was least prepared for it:

> My pregnancy was not planned. I did not want a baby just yet. I am not emotionally ready to take on the responsibility of another baby. My husband uses a sheath so I could not do anything myself to prevent this pregnancy. I suppose I am now resigned to it.
>
> (Gujarati mother, third pregnancy)

It is evident that some of the Gujarati women had accidentally become pregnant. However, in the case of others, pregnancy was not exactly an accident because some were using the contraceptive pill before they conceived. Their comments implied that there was some disagreement between the couples about starting a family. It would appear that in most cases the partner who was most keen to have a baby had either overcome resistance by persuasion or, in some extreme cases, had ignored the objections from the other partner:

> To tell you the truth, it was not planned. At least I was not ready to have a baby. I was a bit disappointed; I suppose I am a career woman . . . I am very ambitious. For my husband it is the right time to have a baby because he is 31 and the right age to become a father. Initially he was worried about my reaction because he knew I was not too keen to have a baby.
>
> (Gujarati mother, first pregnancy)

Such remarks made by some of the first-time mothers suggested that it would be wrong to assume that first-time married mothers have less problems adjusting to their unplanned pregnancies than women who do not want any further additions to their family. The mixed views expressed by some Gujarati women who were expecting their first babies seemed contradictory in the face of strong cultural pressure for them to have a baby soon after marriage. However, it is important to recognize that the younger generation of Asian women may have different interests and aspirations which may conflict with having a baby. Indeed, the reported marked increase in labour market participation rates among educated Asian women, notably the Gujarati Hindu and Punjabi Sikh women, would suggest that their greater economic independence had given them greater negotiating power over their lives, including when to start a family (see, for example, Bhachu 1988).

Although in a majority of the unplanned pregnancies husbands appeared to be more determined to start a family than their wives, there were some exceptions. For example, some women from both communities, albeit few, who were anxious to have a baby had made a unilateral decision to stop using the contraceptive pill without the knowledge of their husbands:

> My pregnancy was half planned. I decided it was the right time for us to have a baby so I just came off the pill. We did not plan it together. He was not keen to have a baby because we had been married for just over a year. But for me it is nothing like having your own otherwise you miss out a lot. When he first found out I was pregnant he was not overjoyed but later he got used to the idea.
>
> (Gujarati mother, first pregnancy)

The greatest anomaly was found where neither partner wanted a further addition to their family nor wished to take the responsibility of birth control:

> We had not taken any precautions because I did not want to carry on taking the pill and I was not keen to have a coil fitted. My husband felt it was my responsibility and he was not prepared to use anything himself. When I became pregnant it took us a long time to come to terms with it. I even considered having an abortion but my doctor persuaded me against it.
>
> (Gujarati mother, third pregnancy)

Another Gujarati woman also cited a similar reason for her mixed attitudes towards her unplanned pregnancy. In her case too, her husband did not think it was his responsibility to prevent a pregnancy:

> After we were married I was on the pill but after my first baby was born I came off the pill because there was such a lot of talk about cancer. My husband did not want me to stop the pill but he was not prepared to use any contraceptive himself. When I became pregnant for the second time it did not matter because we wanted another baby but this time round it is different as neither of us wanted another baby.
> (Gujarati mother, third pregnancy)

Although these were extreme cases, the experiences of these Gujarati women suggest that couples who appear to be fully knowledgeable about family planning and were positively inclined towards the ideas of family spacing and smaller family still experienced a great deal of tension. In both cases the tension existed because the husbands did not see family planning as a shared responsibility. It would seem that the ambiguous attitudes towards fertility control were not related to their lack of interest in family planning but rather their inability to resolve who should take responsibility for birth control. The result of this conflict between the couples was an unwanted pregnancy which had a more immediate impact on the lives of the women than of their husbands.

Bangladeshi couples who were not practising any birth control on religious grounds appeared to be free of the tension experienced by the Gujarati couples. In fact, the comments made by some Bangladeshi women suggested that the locus of control was not with the individual man or woman but was believed to be in the hands of 'Allah': 'I was not very surprised to become pregnant. My husband and I believe that pregnancy is a gift from Allah so we do not mind having children. We must accept the consequences of pregnancy' (Bangladeshi mother, seventh pregnancy).

However, it is important to stress that these views were not shared by all Bangladeshi women, particularly those who were concerned about the effect of an unwanted pregnancy on their health and those who were keen to follow their careers: 'Now if everything goes well this pregnancy, I would like to go back on the pill . . . I have just graduated from the law school and I want to establish my own practice' (Bangladeshi mother, second pregnancy).

## Initial feelings and reactions: coming to terms with pregnancy

Popular images of pregnancy and motherhood create an impression that it is what most women desire and it is their most important achievement in life (Phoenix *et al.* 1991). The idealization of pregnancy also encourages unrealistic expectations of pregnancy. Wolkind and Zajicek (1981), for example, point out that much of the earlier theories and research literature gave credence to idealized notions of pregnancy and motherhood by placing greater emphasis on positive aspects while minimizing or glossing over the negative aspects of pregnancy and their consequences for the lives of women. A more realistic assessment of women's attitudes towards pregnancy and motherhood has begun to emerge from studies which reveal the huge disparity between women's actual experiences and the impression generally given. For examples, the findings of Cartwright (1976), Graham (1977) and Oakley (1979), among others, suggest that, irrespective of social class or parity, it is not uncommon for women to go through a period of uncertainty about having a baby. Evidence also suggests that ambivalent attitudes towards pregnancy persist despite the fact that contraceptives offer women greater control over their fertility (Cartwright 1976; Oakley 1979).

The way women feel and react to their pregnancy has implications for how they manage the transition to motherhood. It is now widely accepted that it is not unusual for pregnant women to experience a full spectrum of emotions ranging from positive to ambivalent to negative feelings about their pregnancy. In most cases negative feelings are confined to the early months of pregnancy and only in a small number of cases do these feelings persist beyond the birth of the baby. They are often associated with a variety of physical and psychological changes that are taking place in the body and the expression of such feelings is a way of resolving conflicts and coming to terms with the prospect of motherhood.

Despite the strong social and cultural pressure for Asian women to have children, the experiences of Gujarati and Bangladeshi women suggest that their reactions to pregnancy are not unlike those reported for women in the white community. When the women from the two communities were asked to describe how they and their husbands felt when they first found out about their pregnancies, their responses ranged from happiness, to considerable doubt and resentment, to total acceptance of pregnancy as God's will.

A majority of women from both communities who had intended to have a baby expressed positive feelings when they realized that they were pregnant. These included many first-time mothers as well as women who wanted an addition to their family. For a Bangladeshi mother having another baby had a special significance:

> I am very pleased. My husband is also very happy I am pregnant. We wanted another baby because I lost my last baby. I was on the pill before I became pregnant with my fifth baby. Because I did not know that once I was pregnant I had to stop taking the pill my baby died when I was eight months pregnant. This is going to be our last baby . . . we both want a boy. We hope we are lucky this time.
>
> (Bangladeshi mother, sixth pregnancy)

It was interesting to observe that considerably more husbands were happy about the pregnancy than were their wives. This marked difference in the attitude towards pregnancy suggests that the pregnancy had a more immediate negative impact on the lives of the women than it had on the lives of the men. This was certainly the case with many Gujarati women, who described their feelings in terms of entrapment and the loss of opportunities to return to paid employment or visit relatives abroad. Comments made by a number of multiparous Gujarati women suggested that coping with their negative feelings about their unplanned pregnancy without the sympathy and support of their husbands was a very distressing experience:

> I was not happy at all. In the beginning I became very depressed and withdrawn. Until I was over two months pregnant I did not tell anyone about my pregnancy so no one knew why I was so depressed. I did not want a third baby because I would have liked to have gone out to work and enjoyed some freedom from home. My husband did not mind having another baby, in fact he is very happy about my third pregnancy. He does not really understand why I am so upset.
>
> (Gujarati mother, third pregnancy)

Although a majority of Bangladeshi women accepted their pregnancies with equanimity, a small number were upset because they had become pregnant sooner than they had expected and were also concerned about the effect on their health:

> I was not very happy at first because I am worried about my health. The doctor at the hospital had told me that I should not become pregnant for two or three years because I had a Caesarean operation. My husband was also anxious at first but now he is happy. He wants a nice boy.
>
> (Bangladeshi mother, second pregnancy)

It was apparent that couples who had not managed to resolve their differences about which partner should take responsibility for contraception faced considerable mental anguish in coming to terms with an unwanted pregnancy. While the lack of control over fertility caused unhappiness to both partners, it had far more serious implications for women:

> We hadn't planned to have a third baby. My husband was not at all pleased. He wanted me to get rid of it. It was quite a difficult time for me because, you know, in my own mind I did not want to do anything bad but there was no choice. My husband was most unhelpful . . . at night he would tell me to arrange a termination and in the morning he would change his mind about termination. I felt trapped from both sides; getting termination was difficult on the NHS and private termination was too expensive.
>
> (Gujarati mother, third pregnancy)

The above example highlights the difficulties faced by some women who were not able to seek emotional and practical support from their immediate families. In dealing with sensitive and emotive issues such as the termination of a pregnancy, family members may not be the most suitable people to provide unbiased advice. It is therefore important to recognize that not all Asian women have support from their extended families when they are faced with difficult decisions of this kind and their attempts to obtain professional advice may not be taken seriously:

> When I found out I was really pregnant I was really worried. I spoke to my doctor and told her that we weren't happy about having this baby and would like to arrange a termination. The doctor told me to try some gin. I don't know if she said that jokingly to cheer me up because I was so depressed. Anyway I was so desperate I took a whole bottle of gin hoping I would lose the baby but nothing happened. I then took a lot of Indian herbal remedy hoping I would miscarry but nothing happened. In the end I just had to accept that there was nothing I could do . . .
>
> (Gujarati mother, third pregnancy)

Evidence from a recent study of Asian parents caring for children with sickle cell and thalassaemia reported similar lack of support and understanding from health professionals (Atkin *et al.* 1998).

The majority of women who expressed doubts and resentment about their pregnancies were Gujarati women who did not want further additions to their family or wanted longer gaps between children. However, negative feelings were not confined to multiparous women as many women expecting their first babies, particularly Gujarati women, expressed misgivings about their pregnancies:

> I was most definitely not ready for a baby. My husband is the eldest male so my parents-in-law were very anxious for us to have a baby. When I became pregnant my in-laws were obviously very pleased. Sometimes I really regret becoming pregnant . . . would have liked to have waited until I was established in my career.
>
> (Gujarati mother, first pregnancy)

## Summary

Some of the main issues to emerge from this chapter suggest that both Gujarati and Bangladeshi women's perceptions of conception were strongly influenced by their cultural and religious attitudes towards marriage, motherhood and the importance of having male children. Although some, particularly Gujarati women, had lived in Britain for a number of years and had adopted western attitudes towards family planning, they all shared the common view that conception should only take place within the institution of marriage.

Allowing for the influence of cultural and religious traditions, it was evident from the accounts of Gujarati and Bangladeshi women that in many respects their experiences were similar to women in the white community.

The similarities in experiences were most apparent in relation to their attitudes towards conception and the inherent ambiguity in planned and unplanned pregnancies. Of the two groups of women, Gujarati women appeared more favourably inclined towards contraception because it provided possibilities to delay having a baby, to determine the gap between pregnancies and to limit the size of the family. The use of contraception was also seen by Gujarati women as offering greater control over fertility to fit in with personal aspirations, including employment. However, in practice, only a small number of women were able to make independent decisions about whether to have a baby or prevent an unwanted pregnancy.

The conflicts women faced in coming to terms with their pregnancies were most evident among women who wanted to delay starting a family and those whose preference for small family size clashed with the pressure to produce a male child. For some women the unresolved dilemma about birth control and which partner should take the responsibility for using contraception created difficulties in their marriage and deeply affected the way they felt about their pregnancies.

For a majority of Bangladeshi women the timing of conception seemed to be less of an issue, as a number of women had recently settled in Britain and their views were still strongly influenced by the cultural and religious traditions of the country of their birth.

Finally, the women's attitudes to birth control and the control over fertility have implications for their subsequent attitudes and behaviour towards the management of their pregnancies and childbirth. A majority of women who did not intend to become pregnant became either resigned or more positive as their pregnancies advanced. However, a small number from both groups who wanted to delay starting a family or who did not want more children continued to experience difficulties in coming to terms with their pregnancies right up to and, in some cases, after the birth of their baby. The resentment which the women felt about their pregnancies became apparent in the interactions they had with other members of the family and in decisions about the management of pregnancy and childbirth. The issue of control and its implications for the management of pregnancy will be addressed in the next chapter.

## Annotated bibliography

Although there is a large volume of literature on the use of contraceptives among South Asian women, there are few examples of in-depth explorations of South Asian women's attitudes to pregnancy. The following collection of papers provides some useful insight.

Atkin, K., Ahmad, W.I.U. and Anionwu, E.N. (1998) Screening and counselling for sickle cell disorders and thalassaemia: the experiences of parents and health professionals, *Social Science and Medicine*, 47(11): 1639–51.

Although this paper is not about women's experiences of pregnancy, the paper includes a discussion of the dilemma mothers face when considering termination of pregnancy when carrying a child with thalassaemia. They report that although cultural and religious beliefs were important considerations, parents' responses to termination were complex and variable.

Woollett, A., Dosanjh-Matwala, N. and Hadlow, J. (1991) The attitudes to contraception of Asian women in East London, *British Journal of Family Planning*, 17: 72–7.

In this paper, Woollett and her colleagues explore Asian women's attitudes to contraception and family building and family spacing. The discussion focuses on the reproductive strategies women use in relation to family building and family spacing.

# 4

# The management of pregnancy

## Introduction

The status of a woman during the gestation period is ambiguous, depending on whether or not her condition is regarded as normal. In non-industrialized societies pregnancy is more likely to be considered as a normal life event and is not treated like an illness which requires expert medical supervision (Oakley 1977; Lozoff *et al.* 1988), although the degree to which it is medicalized may depend on residence in rural and urban locations and social class. For example, in countries such as India and Pakistan, western medicine as well as 'eastern medicine' based on *Unani, Ayurvedic* and *Sidha* exist side by side but the quality and access to care varies between rural and urban locations and the choice is limited by people's ability to pay (Ahmad 1992).

A majority of people live in rural areas where medical care, particularly maternity care, is less well organized and even today in some countries, for instance in rural Bangladesh, India and Pakistan, pregnancy and childbirth are managed by experienced informal practitioners such as *dais* (traditional birth attendants) and experienced older female relatives whose expertise comes not from medical knowledge but from practice and skills passed on from one generation to the next (Blanchet 1984; Jeffery *et al.* 1989). It is often older experienced female relatives, usually a mother-in-law or mother, who take upon themselves the responsibilities of advising and supporting a pregnant mother from the early signs of pregnancy up to childbirth and beyond.

Any dangers to the health and well-being of the pregnant mother and her unborn child are safeguarded against by observation of certain rituals such as ceremonies to appease ancestral spirits (Raja 1993) including observation of both prescriptions and restrictions in the diet or behaviour of pregnant women (Homans 1980; MacCormack 1982). For example, in India and Pakistan beliefs about 'hot' and 'cold' are closely associated with health and illness and are based on the *Ayurvedic* and *Unani* systems of medicine which in their turn are derived from the humoral theory developed by the Greeks (Bhopal 1986; Ahmad 1992). According to this system, the four humours, blood, phlegm, yellow bile and black bile, are possessed by all individuals and they determine the temperament and overall well-being of individuals. Each humour is associated with a unique property or 'temperament': for instance, blood is considered to be hot and moist; phlegm is cold and moist; yellow bile is hot and dry and black bile is cold and dry. Ill health is caused when the balance between the four humours is disturbed. Similar humoral properties of 'hot' and 'cold' are also attributed to symptoms or illnesses as well as to food items and medications. For example, certain conditions such as pregnancy are considered to be 'hot' as are certain foods such as ginger, chilli, dates, nuts, eggs and red meat. 'Hot' conditions need to be balanced by cold foods or behaviour modification to restore the body into a state of equilibrium. Appropriate care during pregnancy therefore requires careful diet and behaviour.

Similar beliefs about 'hot' and 'cold' in relation to post-partum care are discussed more fully in Chapter 6. Evidence from literature suggests that beliefs about 'hot' and 'cold' are also a part of traditional medical systems in countries as far apart as China (Pillsbury 1978; Koo 1984) and many countries in South America (Messer 1981). It is also interesting to note from the broad conclusion drawn by Pillsbury (1978), Homans (1980) and Dobson (1988) and confirmed by my own findings that many practices based on the traditional model of managing pregnancy and childbirth have survived the impact of urbanization and migration across continents despite relatively easy access to western medical care.

This is in direct contrast to the way pregnant women in western industrialized societies are treated (Arms 1975; Oakley 1976; Haire 1978). In Britain, medical professionals have taken over the traditional role of women as providers of care and support for pregnant women. The trend towards the medicalization of childbirth started after the First World War in an attempt to reduce the high incidence of infant and maternal mortality (Oakley 1976). Currently, the medicalization of childbirth begins before conception and gains power in the early weeks of pregnancy. Any woman who suspects that she is pregnant is expected to notify her general practitioner who makes arrangements for antenatal care and hospital delivery. After the pregnancy is confirmed all pregnant women are expected to present themselves at their local clinic or maternity hospital for regular examinations to detect any abnormality or complication. In addition, women are encouraged to attend antenatal preparation classes and follow dietary and health advice given by health professionals (Stacey 1988: 237).

Many women of South Asian origin who have settled in this country encounter, some for the very first time, a totally different system of managing pregnancy and childbirth. This is particularly the case if the childbearing women, or their older female relatives, are familiar with non-medical female-centred childbirth practices. The following accounts of Gujarati

Hindu and Bangladeshi Muslim women provide opportunities to explore cultural differences in the management of pregnancy. Secondly, and more significantly, they provide an opportunity to examine strategies used by women to negotiate two opposing models of care during pregnancy.

Although many features of the traditional model of care during pregnancy are common to Gujarati and Bangladeshi women, the way women approach their care in pregnancy may be influenced by structural differences such as socio-economic position, the length of settlement in Britain, educational attainment and environmental factors such as rural or urban backgrounds. At a personal level, differences in attitudes to care during pregnancy may include the strength of identification with traditional practices, the role and influence of older female relatives and attitudes to the involvement of medical professionals in the management of the pregnancy.

Each of the above factors can have an important bearing on the decisions a woman makes during her pregnancy, starting with the confirmation of the pregnancy, decisions regarding health and diet, antenatal care and the observation of traditional rituals surrounding pregnancy. The ways in which Gujarati and Bangladeshi women managed their care during pregnancy were analysed to explore the relationship between attitudes to traditional and medical models of care.

## Confirmation of pregnancy

If conception has occurred, it is signalled by the absence of the monthly period unless a woman has some other serious illness. A woman who is attuned to her bodily functions may suspect her pregnancy long before anyone else becomes aware of it. Some women have additional symptoms of pregnancy such as sickness, tiredness and dizzy spells which make the pregnancy more obvious.

In cultures where pregnancy and childbirth are not medicalized, less emphasis is placed on the need to have a pregnancy confirmed by a health professional – the symptoms experienced by the pregnant woman would be sufficient proof of her pregnancy. She would then be advised and supported by older female relatives or by a *dai* (traditional midwife) about appropriate diet and behaviour during pregnancy (Blanchet 1984; Jeffery *et al.* 1989). Among the women interviewed, their eagerness to recognize and acknowledge the early symptoms of their pregnancies appeared to be affected by their attitudes towards conception. For example, women who were expecting to become pregnant were more eager to accept the symptoms as a sign of pregnancy whereas women who had not intended to become pregnant were less eager to acknowledge the symptoms that they were experiencing.

More than half the women interviewed claimed that they suspected that they might be pregnant after missing their first period. A small number of women from both groups claimed that they knew instinctively, even before they had missed their period, and a few women reported that their mothers-in-law or other female relatives had suspected that they were pregnant long before their pregnancy was confirmed by their doctor: 'I did not want to believe that I could be pregnant but my sister-in-law suspected that I was pregnant' (Bangladeshi mother, second pregnancy).

Not all women immediately wanted to believe that the symptoms they had experienced had anything to do with pregnancy. This was particularly the case with the women who hoped it was a false alarm: 'At first I was upset and shocked . . . I prayed for the test to be negative. We had not planned to have a baby until we were financially secure. We have just bought our flat . . . pregnancy was the last thing on my mind' (Gujarati mother, first pregnancy).

The organization of maternity services and the treatment of pregnancy as a medical condition require women to obtain medical confirmation of their pregnancy either through their own doctors or through a chemist. This practice was sometimes interpreted by older female relatives as one which usurped their role and devalued their wisdom and experience. In some cases, the negotiation between the traditional and medical management of pregnancy became problematic from the onset of pregnancy. A number of Gujarati Hindu women reported that their relationships with their mothers-in-law were affected because they, the pregnant women, attached greater importance to medical expertise and professional opinion rather than to the opinions of an older female relative:

> My mother-in-law was the first person to remark that I might be pregnant because she had noticed that I was feeling a bit dizzy and nauseous in the morning. I couldn't believe that my mother-in-law was right because the test done by my doctor was negative. My mother-in-law had no doubts that I was pregnant. She felt that bed rest was unnecessary, as the symptoms I was experiencing were common in pregnancy.
>
> (Gujarati mother, first pregnancy)

Since most women in Britain no longer have the choice of giving birth at home, women who are not keen to receive antenatal care still need to see their doctors to reserve a bed in hospital for delivery and obtain certificates which would enable them to claim maternity benefits. It has been widely reported that many Asian mothers fall into the high-risk category during the antenatal period because they do not take full advantage of maternity services (Barnes 1982; Clarke and Clayton 1983). One of the main aims of the Asian Mother and Baby Campaign (launched in 1984) was to urge Asian mothers to report their pregnancies as soon as possible to increase the uptake of antenatal care.

Evidence from the study suggested that there was a wide variation in the length of time women had taken to report their pregnancies to their doctors. The most striking differences were between Gujarati and Bangladeshi women with all but two Gujarati women having their pregnancies confirmed by the 8th week of pregnancy, while a majority of Bangladeshi women had their pregnancies confirmed after the 12th week of pregnancy and a few after the 17th week of pregnancy. The marked difference in the length of time for confirmation of pregnancy among Gujarati and Bangladeshi women is examined here to offer some explanations for this apparent difference. Clearly, persuading Asian mothers to conform to the requirements of health professionals depends, first, on the importance they attach to the medical confirmation of pregnancy, second, on the ease of access to services and third, on what they believe would ensue from reporting their pregnancies.

The Gujarati women seemed to be very keen to have their pregnancies confirmed as soon as possible. The fact that the majority of the Gujarati women were registered with female doctors may have been an important factor in this decision, although some reported that they felt equally at ease with male doctors. In a small number of cases, Gujarati women seemed to place greater faith in their doctors than in their own intuition:

> After I missed my period I did the home pregnancy test. We did the test twice and each time we had a positive result but we still doubted ourselves thinking we couldn't read the test correctly. I went to my doctor to have it confirmed and when he confirmed it then I was sure.
>
> (Gujarati mother, first pregnancy)

Some Gujarati women who had not planned to become pregnant were just as anxious to consult their doctor to allay their fears of an unwanted pregnancy:

> I saw my doctor straight away, as soon as I missed my period. I had gone to my doctor in a way to confirm that I wasn't really pregnant – in my mind I kept saying I wasn't pregnant . . . My husband had also suggested that if the doctor confirmed the pregnancy, I should get something from the doctor to get rid of the baby.
>
> (Gujarati mother, third pregnancy)

In contrast, Bangladeshi women were far more reluctant to seek medical confirmation of pregnancy. A possible explanation for the late reporting by Bangladeshi women may have been the belief that pregnancy was a natural occurrence, which did not require medical intervention. However, it appears that the women's reasons for delaying reporting their pregnancies were more complex. Many revealed in the interviews that they considered hospital births to be safer than home births in rural villages in Bangladesh. Homans's (1980) study of Asian women reports similar findings.

Some Bangladeshi women found it acutely embarrassing to seek a consultation with a male doctor, especially if the doctor was a member of their own community, because they were concerned about breaking the modesty restrictions.

> I became pregnant sometime in October but I did not want to see my doctor because he is Bangladeshi. Although I have been registered with him for the past four years I have not consulted him once. I find it very

> embarrassing to talk to him about my pregnancy. My husband went to see him instead to get a letter for the hospital appointment. I did not see anyone about my pregnancy until I had an appointment at the hospital in January when I was three months pregnant.
>
> (Bangladeshi mother, fifth pregnancy)

Evidence suggests that for many Muslim women the preservation of modesty or 'purdah' is an important issue but is not taken seriously by those who do not share similar cultural practices (Currer 1986; Schott and Henley 1996). Even though the purdah restriction is somewhat relaxed in Britain, many women found it unacceptable to seek consultation with any male doctor. For many Bangladeshi women there was a tension between the desire to gain access to maternity services which they perceived as western and superior, and the cultural need to avoid contact with the opposite sex so as not to violate the purdah restriction.

Even where women had put aside their inhibitions about contact with the opposite sex, for some of them reporting a pregnancy early meant regular attendance at the antenatal clinic, coping with communication difficulties, having to rely on their husbands to accompany them to the clinic and coping with childcare problems. For some of these reasons, women left it as long as possible to confirm their pregnancies. This trend seemed to be quite common among women who had previous experience of antenatal care in Britain:

> I went to see my doctor after I was four months pregnant, although I was quite sure about my pregnancy. The delay to see the doctor was mainly waiting for my husband to be free so that he can be with me and my other children. I have no relatives in this country who can help to look after my children.
>
> (Bangladeshi mother, third pregnancy with history of high blood pressure)

Another Bangladeshi woman intimidated by previous encounters with maternity care in this country was anxious to avoid the encounters as long as it was possible:

> I waited three months before I sent my husband to get a letter for a hospital appointment from my family doctor. I did not want to tell anyone that I was pregnant because I didn't want to go too early . . . if you go too early to your doctor then you have to keep too many appointments. Once I have been given an appointment I do not like to miss it because if you miss any appointments they [doctors] don't like it and ask too many awkward questions.
>
> (Bangladeshi mother, fifth pregnancy)

For many women confirmation of pregnancy was both a cultural and an individual issue. The issue confronting Bangladeshi women was tied up with the fact that they are a recent immigrant group and thus less well acculturated to British expectations about managing pregnancy. In Britain they were suddenly having to deal with another set of expectations. The discussion above throws some light on how they coped with the culturally alien concept of the medical confirmation of pregnancy and how they circumvented consultations with male doctors to preserve their modesty.

In contrast, Gujarati women were more at ease with the medical model of care. However, the personal circumstances of individual women determined whether the confirmation of pregnancy became an issue. The fact that many Gujarati women had lived in Britain over many years and were also accustomed to living in large urban centres gave them an advantage over Bangladeshi women who were relatively new to Britain and more accustomed to living in rural areas. In addition, the Gujarati women's higher socio-economic and educational status made it a lot easier for them to negotiate their care within the health services.

## Perception of health in pregnancy

The issue of pregnancy as a state of normality or ill health has been debated extensively in the literature with opposite views being put forward by the researchers in the field. For instance, Hern (1971) asserts that pregnancy should be treated as ill health whereas Mckinlay (1972) argues that pregnancy should be treated as a normal biological event in the lives of most women which is necessary for the survival of the species. However, for many women such theoretical debate does not match the reality of their experiences.

The way pregnant women view their health in pregnancy is based on subjective experience, coloured by their social and personal circumstances, as well as by the way the pregnancy is defined in cultural terms. Most women do not equate pregnancy *per se* with ill health, although pregnancy is associated with a certain amount of discomfort caused by minor ailments. In addition, how a woman perceives her health in pregnancy depends on her state of health before becoming pregnant.

A majority of women from both communities claimed that they had enjoyed good health before they became pregnant. Gujarati women who had suffered from poor health before their pregnancy described it as a form of emotional and physical exhaustion. They identified a number of reasons for such exhaustion including lack of support with childcare responsibilities, difficult relationships with husbands and in-laws and housing problems. Gujarati women who felt unable to exercise control over their fertility claimed that they were physically and emotionally drained and were unprepared to cope with another pregnancy: 'I felt very depressed and cried a lot. I felt very miserable. My husband is away from home a lot. I was not keeping well after the birth of my first son who just had his first birthday. I was not in a fit state to have another baby but what could I do . . . ?' (Gujarati mother, second pregnancy).

Bangladeshi women who were concerned about their health before they became pregnant often linked their poor health to housing problems and the racism that they encountered in their daily lives:

> I did not feel well . . . I felt very depressed before my pregnancy. Our situation is not good. We have two rooms for all of us in this hotel. The English lady who comes to clean the hotel is rude to us . . . she takes advantage of us because we can't speak English.
>
> (Bangladeshi mother, seventh pregnancy)

The majority of Bangladeshi women were relatively new to this country; it was not surprising that alienation, isolation and poor housing contributed to their lack of well-being. However, evidence gathered from documentary analysis of hospital medical records revealed that many of them also had a history of serious health problems such as high blood pressure and anaemia. From their accounts it was evident that many of them were unaware of their conditions even though their records showed that they were receiving treatment: 'I have no illness apart from morning sickness . . . My health is quite good' (Bangladeshi mother, third pregnancy with a history of high blood pressure).

The apparent discrepancy in the perceptions of health suggested either that these women had different views of good health (see, for instance, Donovan 1986) or more importantly that health professionals failed in communicating the information concerning the seriousness of their condition to the women. The issue of poor access to the medical practitioners raised earlier in the chapter clearly has further implications for women who have serious health problems before they become pregnant. In some women the physiological changes associated with pregnancy may exacerbate health problems which existed before the pregnancy, putting both the mother and her baby at risk. Since the potential risks of high blood pressure, diabetes, anaemia and heart disease are well established, the failure of health professionals to share this information with women from different cultural and linguistic backgrounds, who are also unfamiliar with the western medical care system, places them at unnecessary risk.

In the course of their pregnancies, a third of the women interviewed had experienced some serious health problems with blood pressure, anaemia or depression. Bangladeshi women seemed to be at greater risk, perhaps due to their lower socio-economic position; they also faced added difficulties in gaining access to antenatal care. A Bangladeshi woman with a history of high blood pressure and previous eclamptic fits remarked: 'Although I was quite sure about my pregnancy, I didn't go to my doctor until I was four months pregnant because there is no one to look after my children. I usually have to wait until it is possible for my husband to take me to the doctor' (Bangladeshi mother, third pregnancy).

This particular mother was at risk throughout her pregnancy and was admitted to hospital on two occasions to stabilize her dangerously high blood pressure.

Unlike the Bangladeshi women, Gujarati mothers appeared to be aware of the risk of high blood pressure and anaemia and did not hesitate to seek medical advice. Their greater familiarity with the medical system and family support at home made it easier to maintain control over their health:

> I was very anaemic just when I became pregnant. I was put on iron tablets which helped a lot. Now I have got high blood pressure and swollen ankles and swollen hands. I have been told to rest as much as possible . . . I usually have a nap in the afternoon and put my feet up as much as I can to keep my blood pressure down.
>
> (Gujarati mother, first pregnancy)

The main conclusion to be drawn from the above discussion is that women who had not been influenced by the western medical model of childbirth management believed that a pregnancy was a normal physiological occurrence. As a result it was not surprising that these women, and Bangladeshi women in particular, did not perceive high blood pressure and severe anaemia as a potential threat to their pregnancy. The fact that some of these women were unaware of the seriousness of their state of health has implications for the management and treatment of serious conditions. It also has implications for how information is conveyed to women whose first language is not English.

On the other hand, the accounts of women who were unhappy or worried during pregnancy suggest that the extent to which their emotional problems were linked to social deprivation may not have been fully appreciated by medical professionals. It is important to realize that women whose first language is not English may not be able to voice their concerns adequately to obtain appropriate advice and information.

## Minor ailments in pregnancy

It has been reported that all women regardless of cultural background experience some level of discomfort during pregnancy (Homans 1980, 1985b). However, different cultures have evolved different methods of coping with them. Fortunately most discomforts are transitory and do not cause any serious harm to the mother or the baby, though women may need support and advice to cope with them. In spite of the fact that the majority of the women interviewed claimed that they enjoyed good health in pregnancy, and these also included women who had some serious health problems, almost all experienced a certain amount of discomfort as a result of physiological changes taking place in their bodies. However, not all women were affected to the same degree, and often the extent of discomfort felt in one pregnancy was unique to that particular pregnancy.

Some common minor ailments associated with discomfort in pregnancy are nausea, sickness, tiredness, indigestion, backache, depression, sleeplessness, leg cramps and constipation. Not all women will experience all these problems and some women experience the discomfort in early or late pregnancy whereas others are affected throughout their pregnancies. The majority of the women complained of two or more minor ailments in their pregnancies. The Gujarati women had the largest number of ailments. The commonest ailments were either nausea or sickness which were experienced by almost all women. Other ailments such as tiredness, heartburn, dizzy spells and aches and pains affected almost equal numbers of Gujarati and Bangladeshi women.

## Management of minor ailments in pregnancy

The Gujarati and the Bangladeshi cultures have evolved their own traditional methods of dealing with minor ailments involving the use of certain foods and herbs (Homans 1983, 1985b). In Britain, women from these cultures have an additional method of dealing with minor ailments based on the western allopathic treatment. How an individual woman deals with minor ailments depends on the severity of her complaints and her attitude towards the forms of treatment that are available to her, previous knowledge or experience of the condition, and access to advice and support. Multiparous women who had experienced nausea and sickness in their previous pregnancy claimed that they were psychologically better prepared to cope with it than many first-time mothers: 'Awful! In the beginning it was terrible because of my sickness. I simply hated it . . . In the beginning I was too ill to appreciate the fact that I was pregnant and there was something good about being pregnant. I hadn't expected it to be like this' (Gujarati mother, first pregnancy).

Women who had suffered from sickness or nausea had obtained support from a number of different sources. The Gujarati women took advantage of both the traditional support of their female relatives and the medical support of health professionals to cope with the discomfort caused by nausea and sickness. However, on an individual level, Gujarati women appeared keener to obtain their doctor's opinion. Almost all the Gujarati women had consulted their doctors about their sickness and nausea. A very small number were prescribed anti-sickness tablets and, of these, many made selective use, either not taking them regularly or reducing the prescribed dosage: 'I had very bad sickness until I was over five months pregnant. I was admitted to hospital as my sickness lasted twenty-four hours a day. I was put on sickness tablets. I was supposed to take three tablets but I used to take only one' (Gujarati mother, first pregnancy).

Their relatively easy access to medical services needs to be interpreted with some caution: the majority in the present study were well educated and materially better off, and their situation is not necessarily generalizable to other Gujarati women across the country.

The Bangladeshi women, who tended to have a stoical attitude towards minor ailments in pregnancy, coped with their discomforts as best as they could: 'Sometimes I feel sick . . . But I suppose it's quite normal. I have to just put up with it' (Bangladeshi mother, first pregnancy). However, women expecting their first baby in Britain seemed to be doubly disadvantaged; they were socially isolated and also experienced difficulties negotiating care from the medical services. Because many Bangladeshi families have been fragmented after migration to Britain, the traditional support and advice provided by older female relatives is not available to many women (Katbamna *et al.* 1997). In the absence of such traditional support some women have no choice but to rely heavily on their husbands. While most Bangladeshi husbands take their responsibilities seriously, it is difficult for many husbands to adjust to their new role which requires them not only to give practical support at home but also to negotiate with the health carers. The deep sense of loss expressed by many Bangladeshi women of childbearing age indicates that they have been the main casualties of the break-up of families and social networks: 'I was always feeling sick. Always felt nervous. Sometimes I became crazy to go to my mother's home in Bangladesh. My mother would know how to help me' (Bangladeshi mother, first pregnancy).

It has been suggested by Bangladeshi community workers, interviewed separately for the study, that it is common practice among Bangladeshi Muslim women to take precautions to avoid drawing attention to themselves during pregnancy, or showing any symptoms of pregnancy. It would be socially unacceptable for pregnant women to expose their condition, particularly to the men in the household. However, for many Bangladeshi women, the lack of support from the traditional female-centred social networks meant that they had little choice but to rely increasingly on their husbands for practical support:

> I have no one to give me advice. I have to depend on my husband for everything. This pregnancy I have been feeling very sick all the time. When I could not cope with the sickness I told my husband about it. He managed to get some medicine from our doctor.
>
> (Bangladeshi mother, sixth pregnancy)

Apart from allopathic cures, a number of women resorted to traditional remedies based on assumptions about 'hot' and 'cold' foods and their presumed effect on the body (Homans 1980; Abdulla and Zeidenstein 1982; Dobson 1988; Raja 1993). Since pregnancy is considered as a 'hot' state, symptoms such as sickness or heartburn are treated with cooling foods including some fruits and milk products. Although most of these cures were based on foods and herbs, the remedies recommended by the older experienced women varied from family to family.

A common belief among Bangladeshi women is that the use of tart fruits, such as unripe mango and tamarind, reduces the feelings of nausea and sickness. A number of Bangladeshi women reported that they had eaten sour fruits such as oranges and apples and sometimes sour pickles to get relief from nausea and sickness. Gujarati women were advised to take a mixture of acidic food and spices to control their sickness.

> I was told by my mum to have drops of lemon in water to settle the stomach. My mother-in-law suggested that I should eat a grilled mixture of salt, lemon and cumin which I found very helpful. My doctor also prescribed me some pills but I tried not to take them.
>
> (Gujarati mother, first pregnancy)

However, not all Gujarati women had faith in traditional cures. Some women followed the advice of their female relatives so as not to offend them, as the following remark shows: 'My mother-in-law used to make me a drink from white chalk-like paste to stop the sickness. I had it a couple of times but I didn't believe it would work . . . but I tried it so as not to upset my mother-in-law' (Gujarati mother, second pregnancy).

The ease with which women seek advice and support for other ailments in pregnancy depends on the nature of the ailments and how free they feel about disclosing their complaints to their relatives and the medical professionals. For example, Gujarati women's readiness to seek support from their family members and doctors for sickness and nausea also extended to other ailments, whereas Bangladeshi women continued to rely mostly on their husbands. Although most husbands take their responsibilities seriously some find it difficult to come to terms with their new role. From separate discussion with Bangladeshi community workers, it emerged that many women keep quiet about their ailments because not all husbands are supportive:

> There are two categories of husbands . . . those who are very caring towards their wives throughout their pregnancy and there are those who want their wives to get on with their pregnancy without making a fuss. This causes a lot of extra stress in women . . . some husbands' attitude is that their own mothers managed quite well during their numerous pregnancies in Bangladesh and this attitude leaves some women completely unsupported in this country.
>
> (Bangladeshi Community Social Worker)

Some ailments like tiredness, depression, sleeplessness and aches and pains required sympathetic treatment and physical support, which some women were able to get from their family members. Almost half the women found that discomfort caused by heartburn was just as distressing as sickness and nausea. The women used allopathic cures, traditional cures or both, although more Gujarati women made use of allopathic and traditional remedies than Bangladeshi women. None the less, Gujarati women were often concerned about taking drugs in pregnancy. Medicines prescribed by their doctors were used sparingly and, whenever possible, the women changed their diet to reduce the discomfort: 'My mother-in-law advised me to drink cold milk and to cut down on sour fruits. I also cut down fatty foods from my diet. Although my heartburn did not completely disappear, it made a lot of difference' (Gujarati mother, second pregnancy).

## Anxiety in pregnancy

Evidence from controlled trials suggests that women who lack social and psychological support during pregnancy are more likely to feel unhappy, nervous and worried during pregnancy and more likely to have negative feelings about the forthcoming birth (Elbourne *et al.* 1989). It has also been suggested that pregnancy and childbirth do not necessarily make a woman more vulnerable to depression, but pregnant women whose material and personal circumstances are less favourable are more likely to suffer from anxiety and depression (Brown and Harris 1978; Westwood *et al.* 1989).

Apart from talking about the impact of pregnancy on their physical health, women's accounts also included descriptions of the way pregnancy had affected their emotional stability. In most cases, references to emotional health were interspersed with comments about general health and the women rarely made a distinction between their physical and emotional problems. For some women, the anxiety about a specific physical or emotional problem overshadowed the entire pregnancy and their anxiety appeared as a recurrent theme throughout the interview.

Women gave a variety of reasons for anxiety and depression. For example, women whose personal circumstances were unfavourable or those who were going through an unwanted pregnancy reported that they worried a lot during their pregnancy. The Gujarati women who were unable to prevent their pregnancy were most distressed because they perceived their pregnancy as a trap:

> I have to accept my pregnancy, as there is not much that I can do. I do wonder how I will cope and manage two very young children when my second baby arrives. I am very worried . . . I told my husband that I wanted to arrange an abortion. I was not keeping well and my first baby at the time was only nine months old. I suffered from constant anxiety for the first six months. I was crying all the time. I tried to talk to my husband but he does not listen.
>
> (Gujarati mother, second pregnancy)

The feelings of despair and anxiety were not confined to multipara women who did not wish to be pregnant. A number of Gujarati and Bangladeshi women who were expecting their first babies also expressed similar views. Contrary to expectations, women expecting their first babies were equally worried and unhappy during their pregnancies:

> The first four months were terrible . . . felt down in the dumps. I kept feeling that I shouldn't have become pregnant. I used to be very weepy and felt low. I wouldn't talk to anyone. My in-laws were shocked at my behaviour . . . they were worried. I saw my doctor a couple of times because I was so unhappy but she told me that I wasn't the first woman to experience it.
>
> (Gujarati mother, first pregnancy)

It would also seem from the above comments that if a woman complained about psychological or emotional problems, she was less likely to receive attention than if she complained of physical symptoms. While swings in mood are attributed to hormonal changes, emotional problems which result from unfavourable personal circumstances are often overlooked (Brown and Harris 1978; Graham and Oakley 1981). Often, what may seem a minor problem for some women may cause a great deal of anxiety for others. Sometimes anxiety is expressed in a form which may prevent it from being recognized as such. For example, a number of Bangladeshi women who were housed in temporary accommodation, such as bed and breakfast hotels, complained about headaches and palpitations but their doctors could not find anything wrong with them.

Although the levels of unhappiness expressed by the women in the study varied enormously, their anxiety was not always directly connected with their pregnancy or childbirth. Westwood and colleagues' (1989) study on mental health among Indian and Pakistani women in Leicester revealed that vulnerability to depression was increased by social isolation, poverty, housing problems and the racism encountered by the women in their daily lives. Although MacCarthy and Craissati's (1989) study of stress-related mental disorder in the Bangladeshi community does not make a specific reference to women of childbearing age, it would be surprising indeed if their broad conclusion did not apply equally to women of childbearing age. Many Bangladeshi women in the study reported that adjusting to life in a strange country, separation from relatives and coping with the consequences of being in a lower socio-economic position, such as poor housing, had a far greater effect on their emotional well-being than the thought of being pregnant again. Bangladeshi women who were either living in bed and breakfast hotels or were temporarily housed in council flats while awaiting transfer to more appropriate accommodation were particularly vulnerable to depression:

> I feel anxious all the time . . . I am worried because we have nowhere to live . . . this is temporary. I am not able to relax because I am not used to living in a hotel. It is difficult to look after children and stop them from making noise. My husband is unemployed and it is not easy for him to find a job. Our situation is not good.
>
> (Bangladeshi mother, fourth pregnancy)

While Gujarati and Bangladeshi women shared many anxieties in common with other women in Britain, many of them also had specific concerns about fulfilling the cultural expectations of their reproductive role which heightened their sense of anxiety (see earlier discussion in Chapter 2, page 21). It was evident from the accounts of both groups of women that none of them had been spared from feeling anxious during their pregnancy. Most women had expressed one or more reasons for feeling anxious. Since the first interview took place in the last trimester of pregnancy, anxiety about the forthcoming labour was uppermost in the minds of the women (anxiety concerning forthcoming labour will be discussed more fully in the next chapter). This was especially so among almost all the Gujarati women regardless of their parity. Foetal abnormality or the health of the unborn baby was the next most frequently cited reason for anxiety. A number of Bangladeshi women had added reasons for feeling anxious, as they had lost a baby in the past:

> I am quite worried about my baby and I am thinking if it will happen again. Before this pregnancy my baby was stillborn. It happened when I was eight months pregnant. My doctor told me it was because I had continued taking the pills after I was pregnant. I was very sad, because it was a boy. I am very worried if something should go wrong with this baby.
>
> (Bangladeshi mother, sixth pregnancy)

The anxiety of Gujarati women about the health of their babies could not be linked directly to any previous unfortunate experience. However, it appears that, with two exceptions, their anxiety was in some way related to their ambivalent attitude towards their pregnancies. The women who had an unwanted pregnancy felt that their own negative attitude was having a harmful effect on their unborn baby:

> I am very anxious for the baby. I feel my baby moves uneasily. I am anxious because I wanted to terminate this pregnancy but my doctor persuaded me against termination. I feel the baby must be suffering psychologically because I have such negative attitude towards this pregnancy.
>
> (Gujarati mother, fourth pregnancy)

Another Gujarati woman who had unsuccessfully attempted to abort her baby by taking traditional medicines and consuming a large quantity of alcohol was very worried about having a deformed baby, as her remark suggests:

> This time I have taken so many tablets as well as home made remedies in my early pregnancy. I am really worried they may have done some harm to the baby. The doctor can't tell me anything. I can't even talk to anyone. I will just have to wait and see.
>
> (Gujarati mother, third pregnancy)

After anxiety about foetal abnormality, the next most common cause of anxiety mentioned by the Gujarati and Bangladeshi women was the sex of the baby. In most cases the women's anxiety about the sex of the baby was related to their community's desire for them to produce a male child (see Chapter 3, page 22). Although it would be understandable for a woman who only has daughter(s) to feel under pressure to produce a male child, it became apparent during the follow-up interviews in the postnatal period that the sex of the baby had caused just as much anxiety to women expecting their first child. It is very common for women who fail to produce a male child to blame themselves and consequently, among Hindus, some women observe religious fasts and offer prayers to their family deity in an attempt to conceive a male child.

Although religious teaching among Bangladeshi Muslims does not encourage similar beliefs, male children are desired for economic reasons. They are seen as insurance against old age and as an aid to economic survival. The birth of a male child is greeted with delight; the birth of a female child is considered a liability because, after her marriage, she will belong to her husband's family and will be of no support to her parents. In addition, according to Islamic laws, a man can have more than one wife and, in some interpretations, a man can divorce a wife who fails to bear him a son. The fear of husbands' remarriage induced many Bangladeshi women to undergo repeated pregnancies in order to produce a male child. A mother expecting her fifth baby who had three daughters and one unsuccessful pregnancy was resigned to try again for a boy if her present pregnancy did not result in the birth of a son. Her anxiety was evident in her remarks:

> I have three daughters so this time I hope it will be a boy. I am praying 'Allah' will help me this time . . . My family in Bangladesh are all praying for me to have a boy. My husband is very anxious that we should have a son. I am very much worried and think about the sex of the baby all the time.
>
> (Bangladeshi mother, fifth pregnancy)

Many of the younger generation of Gujarati and Bangladeshi couples in Britain do not share such views. However, cultural beliefs and traditions perpetuated by older members of their respective communities can sometimes cause a lot of mental anguish. In some cases, their husbands are pressurized by relatives to get divorced and remarry.

> My jeth [brother-in-law] has been asking if my husband would find a second wife who will give him a son or would remain a *goolam* [subservient] to me. I feel very inadequate . . . why me? Why could I not have a son?
>
> (Bangladeshi mother, third pregnancy)

Increased family responsibility with the arrival of another baby and housing and financial difficulties were also cited as examples of factors which caused a great deal of anxiety and depression among Bangladeshi and Gujarati women. A Gujarati mother who was expecting another baby very soon after the birth of her first baby commented:

> I don't know how I will manage when the second baby comes. I feel so depressed. My husband does not share my concern. He believes that a young person like me should be able to cope with two young children. I feel emotionally and physically drained. Just the thought of having yet another baby to look after makes me depressed and anxious.
>
> (Gujarati mother, second pregnancy)

A few Bangladeshi women who were waiting to be rehoused found that living in temporary accommodation caused them a great deal of anxiety:

> I feel very depressed sometimes . . . I am worried because my baby is due soon and we are still waiting for a flat. The children and I stay in the rooms all the time because I am afraid to go out anywhere on my own. My husband works in a restaurant and he often comes home late. I can't fall asleep until my husband comes in because I am worried about him.
>
> (Bangladeshi mother, fifth pregnancy)

By way of summary, the Bangladeshi and Gujarati women's anxieties about childbirth and the fear of producing a malformed baby is something they shared with other British women. The cause of these anxieties may be duly acknowledged and receive sympathetic treatment. However, the plight of women who are anxious about the sex of the baby or who are going through pregnancy under difficult personal circumstances may not be fully appreciated by health workers from different cultural and social backgrounds. These factors are ever-present in the lives of many of these women and affect the outcome of their pregnancies and their general health during and after pregnancy.

The accounts of women who were unhappy or worried during pregnancy suggest that the extent of their emotional problems linked to social deprivation may not have been fully appreciated by medical professionals. It is important to realize that women whose first language is not English may not be able to express their anxieties or concerns to health professionals. Health professionals' criticisms, that Asian patients have a tendency to express psychological or emotional distress as physical symptoms, are noted in the literature (Rack 1980).

## Antenatal care in pregnancy

In countries like India and Bangladesh where antenatal care is not organized at the national level, management of pregnancy is traditionally left in the hands of other women. Many pregnant women go through their pregnancy without consulting any medically qualified persons (Blanchet 1984; Jeffery *et al.* 1989). In Britain, antenatal care is provided for all mothers under the National Health Service (NHS). The antenatal care is usually shared between a woman's general practitioner and her local maternity hospital and involves regular medical examination.

For South Asian women who have migrated from countries where antenatal care is only available to those who can afford it, antenatal care offered under the NHS may seem very attractive. However, as the review of the literature (Chapter 2, page 9) suggests, South Asian women often have to overcome numerous physical and psychological barriers to gain access to antenatal care (Clarke and Clayton 1983; Leeds FHSA 1992).

For many Gujarati and Bangladeshi women, having a baby in Britain brings them into contact with health workers from a different social and cultural background. There is strong evidence to suggest that apart from overcoming challenges posed by cultural, language and communication difficulties, factors such as intrusive examination, location of clinics, transport problems and racist attitudes among some medical and nursing staff are not conducive to the take-up of antenatal services (Bowler 1993). However, the findings of the present study broadly confirm evidence from other studies (Dobson 1988; Woollett *et al.* 1995) that, despite the criticism of the quality of care provided, many South Asian women are anxious to receive care. For example, the attendance at antenatal clinics by Gujarati and Bangladeshi women was comparable with other studies on Asian women (Dobson 1988; Woollett *et al.* 1995), with just under a third of women from each group failing to keep all their appointments. The observed difference in the uptake of antenatal care between South Asian women from different subgroups and within each subgroup is a reflection of the enormity of the problems encountered by individual women, and their behaviour is indicative of the limited options they have in negotiating antenatal care.

The accounts of Bangladeshi women suggested that the sex and race of the doctor were also important factors in determining acceptability of antenatal care. About half the Bangladeshi women were receiving all their antenatal care at their hospital antenatal clinic and the rest were receiving shared care from their general practitioners and their local maternity hospital. The Bangladeshi women who were only attending the hospital antenatal clinic were all registered with male Bangladeshi general practitioners. Some of these women had not reported their pregnancies to their family doctors until they were over three months pregnant. The late confirmation of pregnancy by some Bangladeshi women and their preference for hospital-based antenatal care were closely related to their reluctance to be cared for by male doctors who were their countrymen. A majority of Bangladeshi women claimed that they preferred to receive antenatal care at the hospital because they could request to be examined by a female doctor; failing that, white male doctors were preferable to Bangladeshi male doctors. Although these women had no guarantee that a female doctor would see them, they were not put off going to hospital: 'I do not like to go to Dr X because I feel embarrassed . . . he comes from same district . . . he is Bengali like me. Sometimes if I am lucky I see a lady doctor at the hospital' (Bangladeshi mother, fifth pregnancy).

For these women, then, communication difficulties encountered with hospital staff were preferable to breaking purdah restrictions with a male Bangladeshi doctor. The availability of a female Bengali interpreter at the hospital was another factor in some women's preference for attending the hospital antenatal clinic. In contrast, all the women in the Gujarati sample were receiving shared care between their family doctor and the hospital. Gujarati women were in the fortunate position of being able to register with female doctors; two-thirds of Gujarati women were registered with female doctors and half of these were registered with Indian female doctors. Gujarati women who were attending the general practitioners' antenatal clinics were receiving joint care from the community midwives and their family doctors.

Gujarati and Bangladeshi women gave a variety of reasons for missing their appointments. Among Gujarati women, failure to keep appointments seemed to be tied up with feelings of ambiguity towards an unplanned pregnancy; for some, the lack of time coupled with childcare difficulties or pressure to help with the family business took priority over an antenatal appointment: 'I missed some appointments at the surgery because the Wednesday clinic appointments are inconvenient for me to attend. I can't manage to go because I have to help out at our family shop. I missed quite a lot in the beginning' (Gujarati mother, second pregnancy).

The main reasons given by Bangladeshi women for missing appointments were problems with childcare and having to rely on their husbands to escort them to the clinic. Some of these women lacked the confidence to go out on their own because they had been in Britain for less than a year. It was often difficult for some husbands to arrange time off work to accompany their wives to the clinic: 'Yes, I missed some appointments. I don't have anyone to look after my children. My husband has to take time off work to look after my children. It is not always easy for him to take time off from work' (Bangladeshi mother, third pregnancy).

Despite the fact that many Bangladeshi women experienced difficulties attending clinic, their attitude towards antenatal care was very positive.

In short, antenatal care did not pose any problems on cultural grounds for Gujarati women who have been in this country for a number of years, although women's personal circumstances determined the level of uptake of antenatal care. This was particularly evident among women who were unable to exercise control over their fertility.

Bangladeshi women appear to be just as keen to receive antenatal care although their lack of access to female doctors and problems of communication prevented them from making full use of the services available. On a personal level, communication difficulties, relatively recent settlement in Britain and their dependence on male relatives were important factors in determining the level of utilization of antenatal care.

## Diet in pregnancy

An adequate diet is essential for maintaining good health but it assumes even greater significance when a person goes through a vulnerable phase – such as during illness or pregnancy (Homans 1983). The earlier discussion of the management of minor ailments mentioned the use of certain food items by Gujarati and Bangladeshi women. Many cultures have evolved dietary ideologies based on the concept of balancing 'hot' and 'cold' foods and on the restriction of the intake of certain foods to restore the equilibrium of the body. For example, in the Indian subcontinent the notion of 'hot' and 'cold' foods, medicine and conditions stems from the ancient medical system of *Ayurveda* in India and the *Unani* system based on the Greek humoral theory (Bhopal 1986; Raja 1993; Schott and Henley 1996).

Some dietary restrictions and taboos about food, the reasons for which have been lost in the mists of time, have been incorporated into the religious traditions of individual families. Practical knowledge about the inherent properties of certain foods classified as 'hot' or 'cold', and other dietary restrictions in pregnancy, are traditionally passed down the generations through women. Although Gujarati and Bangladeshi women often shared beliefs about 'hot' and 'cold' foods, their dietary habits were governed by different religious practices, education and socio-economic position. The majority of the Gujarati women belonged to the Hindu faith. Hindus believe in the sacredness of all life and therefore the killing of animals is prohibited. Most orthodox Hindu families are lacto-vegetarians, i.e. they avoid eggs, fish, cheese and meat in their diet. A staple vegetarian diet consists of pulses, cereals, milk products and fresh vegetables. However, not all Gujarati Hindu women observe a strict lacto-vegetarian diet as many include cheese and eggs and, occasionally, poultry and mutton.

The Bangladeshi women belonged to the Muslim faith. The staple diet of Bangladeshi families consists of 'halal' meat, fish, rice and vegetables (Schott and Henley 1996). Many classes of animals are not permitted (most scavengers and meat eaters). For meat to be acceptable it must belong to a permitted class of animal and killed appropriately.

Since dietary beliefs in pregnancy are strongly rooted in cultural and religious traditions, we need to address the implications of migration on these dietary beliefs. We also need to look at the role of other members of the family in safeguarding dietary habits in accordance with cultural and religious traditions. In addition, pregnant women have to take on board the dietary advice received from health workers based on western nutritional concepts. Among the Gujarati and Bangladeshi communities in Britain, religious considerations outweigh external pressure to change their dietary beliefs. The need to maintain a strict dietary regime is strongest among the older generation as a way of preserving cultural traditions and identity. The Gujarati women were expected to retain strict vegetarian traditions in the home although similar restrictions did not generally apply to the male members of the family. This often became a cause of conflict for the young generation of women who did not share the values of older members of the family. Gujarati women appeared to be most affected; few Bangladeshi women reported similar concerns about diet: 'My father-in-law has very orthodox views on diet. My father-in-law believes that Indian women should not eat eggs, he therefore wouldn't approve of his daughters-in-law who ate eggs' (Gujarati mother, first pregnancy).

The fact that the present generation of Gujarati women of childbearing age have changed their diet is reflected in their more relaxed attitude towards a non-vegetarian diet, which previously would have been unacceptable on religious and cultural grounds. For example, with the exception of one

Gujarati woman who was strictly lacto-vegetarian, the rest were either not strictly lacto-vegetarians or vegetarians.

After pregnancy, there was no significant change in the dietary habits of the Bangladeshi women, with the exception of minor changes brought about as a result of altered taste. In contrast, there was a noticeable change in the dietary habits of some Gujarati women. Some reported that their diet had changed in a number of ways after becoming pregnant, partly due to changes in taste and partly as a direct result of dietary restrictions enforced by family members in keeping with cultural traditions, as we shall see later. In addition, some women also modified their diet according to advice they received from health professionals.

For example, some Gujarati women claimed they had increased their intake of milk, eggs, cheese and fruit to comply with dietary advice they had received from medical professionals. It is interesting to note that quite a few Gujarati women were prepared to increase their intake of dairy produce, eggs and fruits although they were aware that such advice was contrary to traditional belief. Eggs are considered 'hot' according to the Ayurvedic tradition, besides being an unacceptable source of food for orthodox Hindus as already mentioned. It appears that Gujarati women were sometimes prepared to defy cultural traditions because they felt that by adopting the dietary advice given by medical professionals, they were giving a healthier start to their babies: 'I take more care about what I eat. Doctor told me to take more milk, fruits and vegetables in my diet. I try to drink more milk than I do when I am not pregnant . . . I would not take any notice of what my mother-in-law says. I listen to my doctor' (Gujarati mother, second pregnancy).

Another Gujarati mother, who was very anxious to follow the diet recommended by her doctor, found that she could only do so at the expense of her in-laws' displeasure:

> My doctor told me to increase my intake of milk and eggs because I haven't gained enough weight in my pregnancy. I try and have a pint of milk in my diet. Because my father-in-law has such orthodox views about eggs I can't eat eggs openly so I have one egg a day which I eat secretly in the kitchen. My mother-in-law and my sister-in-law are not very sympathetic because they did not have any problem gaining weight in their pregnancies.
>
> (Gujarati mother, first pregnancy)

For non-vegetarian Bangladeshi women adopting the dietary advice given by medical professionals may not appear to be an issue, and yet none of the Bangladeshi women interviewed mentioned milk, eggs or fruits in their diets. A Bangladeshi community worker reported that dietary advice, which encourages intake of dairy produce, is unacceptable to Bangladeshi pregnant mothers because they dislike the smell and taste of British milk which is not as creamy and rich as the buffalo milk which they drank in Bangladesh.

The fact that Bangladeshi women are non-vegetarian did not mean that they did not have any dietary problems. Since the majority of Bangladeshi women had recently settled in Britain, many of them craved the foods which were indigenous to Bangladesh. Although such food items are available in Britain, they are costly and seasonal, taking them out of the reach of Bangladeshi families on low incomes. Many Bangladeshi women demonstrated a strong association with their cultural traditions in pregnancy by craving the same kinds of foods which pregnant women in Bangladesh are known to crave in pregnancy, such as dried fish *shutki* and tart foods like unripe mango and spicy pickles. In contrast, the type of foods craved by the Gujarati women, particularly younger women, reflected an acquired taste for western foods such as pizza, potato chips and cakes.

Within South Asian communities, older women play a central role in passing down knowledge about family traditions. Older women, by virtue of their age and experience, are vested with the power and authority to instruct younger women in the family about dietary beliefs and to enforce restrictions. Although many Bangladeshi women reported that they were not always able to satisfy their cravings, they appeared to observe fewer dietary restrictions than Gujarati women. The fact that only a small number of Bangladeshi women were living with older female relatives might explain why so few mentioned dietary restrictions. In contrast, a majority of Gujarati women were living in extended households and most had received instructions about an appropriate diet in pregnancy.

Some of the dietary restrictions which women were required to observe related to food considered either too 'hot' or too 'cold' according to *Ayurvedic* and *Unani* concepts. For example, nuts, garlic and ginger were considered to be 'hot' and therefore many Gujarati women reported that they had been advised by their mothers-in-law to avoid eating nuts, ginger and garlic: 'In my early pregnancy I was admitted into hospital because I was feeling very sick. My mother-in-law would not allow me to eat anything on the menu which contained nuts. She told me that it was not good for the baby' (Gujarati mother, first pregnancy).

However, other dietary restrictions connected with religious ritual were not strictly observed. For instance, a few Gujarati women were advised to avoid sesame seeds in their diet in honour of ancestral spirits or the family deity, in the belief that their ancestral spirits would in turn safeguard their passage from pregnancy to childbirth:

> My mother-in-law told me that I should not eat sesame seeds or coconut because it would give offence to our family *devi* [deity]. But I love eating *pan* [stuffed beetlenut leaf] which contains both shredded beetlenut and coconut. She tells me off for being disrespectful to our *devi* and believes that I will have problems in my pregnancy.
>
> (Gujarati mother, fourth pregnancy)

In some cases, dietary restrictions originated from someone in the family having an unfortunate experience and an item of food is avoided in the belief that it was responsible. In interviews where mothers-in-law were present, they explained why their daughters-in-law were asked to avoid certain foods such as sesame seeds and bananas in their diet. One mother-in-law commented:

> We do not eat any sesame seeds in any form during pregnancy. If a woman eats sesame seeds in pregnancy, it [sesame seeds] encourages the growth of the afterbirth at the expense of the baby. The afterbirth leaves no room for the baby to grow in the womb.
>
> (Gujarati mother-in-law)

Sometimes dietary advice given by female relatives conflicted with the advice given by medical professionals:

> It is very confusing – at hospital they tell you to eat nuts and bananas. My mother-in-law tells me to avoid nuts and bananas. My mother-in-law used to advise so many other pregnant ladies and, as she is my mother-in-law, I have to listen to her. You just don't know how to react. I didn't know whom to believe.
>
> (Gujarati mother, first pregnancy)

A number of Bangladeshi women reported that they were advised by their mothers-in-law to avoid pineapple during pregnancy because it is believed to cause miscarriage. The eating of raw pineapple is also associated with abortion of unwanted pregnancies (Abdulla and Zeidenstein 1982). It was also believed that eating pineapples in pregnancy made the baby deformed: 'My mother-in-law said that pineapple is harmful for the baby. She said that pineapples could cause serious damage to the baby's skin in the womb' (Bangladeshi mother, fifth pregnancy).

Of the two groups of women, dietary restrictions in pregnancy had a greater impact on Gujarati women. However, not all Gujarati women were convinced that any harm would come to them or their babies if they disregarded the advice of their mothers or mothers-in-law. Many questioned the rationale behind such restrictions, particularly where the older female relatives were unable to provide adequate explanations. Reactions to restrictions were mixed. Some women who were not convinced about the merit of classifying foods and conditions into 'hot' and 'cold' categories or who had not observed such practices in their natal homes expressed strong reservations and interpreted the imposition of such restrictions as a way of exercising relative autonomy:

> My own mother did not observe any such restrictions because my grandmother forgot to tell her. My mother was quite lucky. I do find it restrictive – especially living in a modern world and in another country and having to observe such restrictions is most inconvenient. It may be that sesame seeds did not agree with a woman and now it is just passed down the line – becoming incorporated into religious beliefs. I must say I don't believe in it.
>
> (Gujarati mother, first pregnancy)

Other women felt that, although they had considerable doubt about the importance attached to dietary practices in the management of pregnancy, it was a small concession to make in order to keep their female relatives happy. Indeed, in taking their relatives' views into account, many women were acknowledging the fact that bringing a child into the family was seen to be a family affair and the advice of others was regarded as entirely legitimate. In some cases, women were not prepared to go against advice in case something went wrong:

> Even if you do go ahead and disregard their advice, and if then something were to happen or you have it at the back of your mind that worry – will something happen now that you have disobeyed? I think it is a stupid theory. My mother-in-law is not the only one; there are other women of the same age group who have told me things I must not eat.
>
> (Gujarati mother, second pregnancy)

Only two Gujarati women were not prepared to dismiss advice based on the accumulated experiences and cultural knowledge of their mothers and mothers-in-law:

> Both my mother and my mother-in-law had five children each, so they know quite a lot about pregnancy. I presume, I mean you have to take some advice from them – there must be some truth in it for them to tell you this. I don't feel badly about having to observe some restrictions.
>
> (Gujarati mother, first pregnancy)

Many mothers-in-law felt that since they had observed the restrictions in good faith in their time, they wanted their daughters-in-law to follow the family tradition. In some cases the imposition of dietary restrictions resulted in a power struggle between older female relatives who tried to impose their views over their daughters or daughters-in-law. Gujarati women not living with their husband's family explained that they were free from such constraints, as they were not under the jurisdiction of their mothers-in-law.

Like people in general, Bangladeshi and Gujarati women, then, come from cultures with well-established concepts which link health with diet, and good health emanates from restoring the physiological state of the body by balancing the diet with 'hot' or 'cold' foods. However, many Asian women of childbearing age in Britain are confronted with the problem of receiving conflicting dietary advice. This tension was particularly apparent with Gujarati women confronted with two different models of care during pregnancy, which required delicate negotiation. Some deployed strategies to circumvent the restrictions without appearing to cause offence. For others, compromise provided the best solution. In contrast, Bangladeshi women appeared not to have this conflict because, as recent immigrants, their identification with their cultural values was still very strong.

## Ceremonial rituals in pregnancy

Apart from the importance of dietary restrictions in the management of pregnancy, ceremonial rituals are integral to the traditional management of care during pregnancy to ensure a safe transition to childbirth. In many cultures around the world where the transition from pregnancy to childbirth is associated with danger, the fear of mishap is overcome by the performance of ceremonial rituals (Kitzinger 1978; Blanchet 1984; McDonald 1987). The observation and performance of such rituals have additional meanings and values attached to them. For example, these rituals accord some privileges to a pregnant woman by marking the significance of her status. These privileges take the form of a greater variety and share of food and less expectation of routine household chores (Pillsbury 1978). Although the rituals in pregnancy and childbirth centre mostly around a pregnant mother, in some cultures the pregnant woman's partner or husband is also required to take part in rituals at the time of birth and in the postnatal period.

Because the transition from pregnancy to childbirth has been made relatively safe as a result of medical advances in antenatal care, as well as the improved socio-economic position of pregnant women and better nutrition and hygiene, some of the rituals performed during pregnancy may seem unnecessary and out of place in modern Britain. The fact that the ceremonial rituals have survived after migration to Britain suggests that observation is crucial for retaining cultural values and identity. In Britain, Gujarati and Bangladeshi women are confronted with two different approaches to safeguarding the transition from pregnancy to childbirth, i.e. ritualization of childbirth versus medicalization of childbirth. Many feminists in the west have argued that medicalization of childbirth is a different form of ritualization (see, for instance, Kitzinger 1978; Oakley 1980). The decision of the women interviewed, about observing rituals, appeared to be determined by how meaningful they found them in a British context where care during pregnancy is based on different principles. The analysis presented here concerns mostly Gujarati women because the interviews with Bangladeshi women failed to generate information on this particular issue. This does not necessarily mean that such rituals have lost their significance within the Bangladeshi community. It is possible that the enactment or performance of rituals requires the presence of well-established social networks of women and material resources. The relatively isolated position of Bangladeshi women in Britain coupled with the lack of well-established female networks and material resources may be reasons for the absence of ceremonial rituals during pregnancy.

Examples of some of the common rituals which formed important aspects of care during pregnancy included the 'Khoro' (lap ceremony), hair washing restrictions in the first seven months of pregnancy, and avoiding contact with other parturient mothers. This subject continues to receive a great deal of attention in the literature suggesting that, despite the passage of time and practical difficulties of organizing these rituals, the performance remains an important part of social life of South Asians in this country (Raja 1993). A number of Gujarati women expecting their first baby reported that they were not allowed to wash their hair for the first seven months of their pregnancy or to come into contact with parturient mothers. Multiparous Gujarati women also claimed that in their first pregnancy they had followed the advice of their mothers-in-law about hair washing and avoiding contact with newly delivered mothers. Thus the customary visit to labour wards offered as a part of the hospital antenatal classes was often not acceptable. Although the restriction on hair washing and the seventh month ceremonial ritual were only observed during the first pregnancy, the restriction on visiting the labour ward by pregnant women was not confined to the first pregnancy: 'I am not allowed to visit anyone who has just had a baby – well at least for four weeks. According to my mother and my mother-in-law it brings bad luck in your pregnancy if you see a newly born baby's face or the face of the baby's mother' (Gujarati mother, second pregnancy).

For some women this restriction was not lifted even if the two women were closely related: 'My brother's wife just had a baby but I am not allowed to visit her until my nephew is over two weeks old. My Narand [husband's sister] stopped me from visiting my brother's wife but I have spoken to her on the phone' (Gujarati mother, first pregnancy).

After the seventh month of pregnancy, a *Khoro* ceremony (filling a mother's lap) is performed in anticipation of the baby's arrival. At the time of the *Khoro* ceremony a woman is required to have a ritual bath and hair wash. During celebration of these rituals a pregnant woman seeks protection from her family deity for a safe delivery. This social occasion also gives the family relations an opportunity to acknowledge the pregnancy. A woman is required to observe this ritual in her first pregnancy only. Immediately after the ceremony, it is common practice among some women to return to their maternal homes for the remainder of their pregnancy and childbirth (Mayor 1984; Blanchet 1984).

The ritual at the seventh month of pregnancy was a common feature among the Gujarati women interviewed. Almost all the Gujarati women expecting their first baby mentioned that they were either expected to participate in this ceremony or had done so in their first pregnancy: 'I had a *Khoro* ceremony at the seventh month of my pregnancy. My mother-in-law had invited a Brahmin [a Hindu priest]. He chanted some holy words to ward off evil spirits and to give me strength and protection for labour' (Gujarati mother, first pregnancy).

Gujarati women had fewer objections to taking part in this ceremonial ritual at the seventh month of pregnancy because it was a social occasion, which conferred on a woman her new status as a mother. Participation in this ritual was also less problematic for women because it could be safely performed within the community and it did not clash with medical management of pregnancy. Consequently most women were eager to participate: 'At the end of the seventh month I had a small *Khoro* ceremony. My in-laws invited immediate family members from both sides of the family. I felt very good about it' (Gujarati mother, first pregnancy).

There is little evidence to suggest that similar ceremonial rituals are important aspects of Bangladeshi culture, although one Bangladeshi mother expecting her first baby mentioned that her family had organized a family celebration in honour of her pregnancy. Clearly, for many women, celebration of their pregnancy was more than a ritual but a public affirmation of their valued status within the family. In fact, women who did not have a *Khoro* ceremony felt most aggrieved, as this remark suggests: 'My mother-in-law doesn't believe in such things. I was expecting to have a ceremony, I must admit. I would have liked to have had it. I was most disappointed' (Gujarati mother, second pregnancy).

However, not all Gujarati women were willing to observe the traditional customs and found other ceremonial rituals restrictive and unnecessary. With the exception of one Gujarati woman who refused to have anything to do with ceremonial rituals, the rest either did so happily or under some duress. A majority of Gujarati women expecting their first babies and who had professional jobs found the restrictions on hair washing most objectionable:

> It's very annoying and irritating. I mean, I find myself asking why would they ask you to do something like this? The only reason I think is to make yourself sexually unattractive to your husband. But living with your in-laws – they put a lot of emphasis on these things and make you feel as if you are a naughty girl . . . I was very annoyed when I was working – holding a managerial position, I did mind what my colleagues thought about my appearance.
>
> (Gujarati mother, first pregnancy)

Other Gujarati women who had expressed similar resentment of the hair washing restriction felt compelled by their female relatives to preserve family traditions. However, Gujarati women who were not living with their in-laws reported that they ignored the instruction of their mothers-in-law:

> When my mother-in-law told me that it was a family custom that daughters-in-law should not wash their hair for the first seven months of pregnancy, I told her that I was going to work and I couldn't go to work without washing it. My Dherani (husband's brother's wife) who is also expecting a baby is not washing her hair because she lives with my mother-in-law. I did ask my mother-in-law the reason behind it but she didn't know. I felt, there was no point to it . . . I was made to feel like an outcast for disobeying.
>
> (Gujarati mother, first pregnancy)

It appears that the tradition of observing ceremonial rituals during pregnancy is deeply rooted, particularly among Gujarati women. Any ceremonial rituals which could be observed within the confines of their own communities created the least problems, and in fact some rituals which proclaimed their pregnant status were most welcome. On the other hand, rituals which could not be observed discreetly, such as the hair washing restriction and the restriction which stopped a pregnant woman going near a parturient mother, resulted in a tension between the women and their older female relatives (see also Drury 1991). The younger women felt that without adequate explanations, such restrictions were meaningless in modern Britain.

## Summary

From the accounts given in the previous chapter, the women from both groups appeared to show that the pattern of managing their pregnancy was deeply rooted in their cultural traditions and was often in sharp contrast to the medically orientated model of managing a pregnancy in Britain. In many aspects of care in pregnancy, women were confronted with two different sets of cultural expectations which made it necessary for the women to negotiate choices. In Britain, hospital delivery is more or less compulsory for most women and antenatal care comes as a package with hospital delivery. When confronted with two different models of care, women from both communities were, where possible, selecting aspects of care to suit their personal circumstances. The decisions of some Gujarati women reflected their more favourable attitudes towards medical care, but the decisions of the majority of Gujarati and Bangladeshi women were based on a compromise between the two systems. It was also evident that women could restrict their contact with medical care to an absolute minimum but could not avoid it altogether.

One of the main points to emerge from the accounts given by Bangladeshi and Gujarati women concerning the management of their pregnancies was that not only were there major differences in the way the Bangladeshi and Gujarati women managed their pregnancies but there were also major differences between individual women. This has implications for not treating all Asian women as if they belong to a single homogeneous group.

There were additional factors which influenced the behaviour of individual Gujarati and Bangladeshi women. Some of these factors were in part related to their attitudes to traditional and medical management of pregnancy and in part to differences in their social and economic status. For instance, the relationship between socio-economic status and utilization of the maternity services reported by Oakley (1984) and Macintyre (1981) could equally apply to Bangladeshi women, many of whom experienced additional disadvantages due to language and communication difficulties and material disadvantages.

Consequently some of the major issues concerning the management of pregnancy centred round the need for the medical confirmation of pregnancy, perceptions of health in pregnancy, antenatal care, diet in pregnancy and the role of ceremonial rituals during pregnancy. For the Bangladeshi women, medical confirmation of pregnancy, concepts of health and illness in pregnancy and antenatal care were major issues because they had to resolve the conflicting expectations of their own cultural beliefs and the lack of familiarity with the medical system. The way some Bangladeshi women coped with this conflict was to delay contact with the medical services as long as possible.

On the other hand, confirmation of pregnancy, antenatal care and potentially conflicting concepts of health and illness in pregnancy were not major issues for the Gujarati women because they had adopted many western values concerning the management of pregnancy. However, because many Gujarati women were living within extended households, their views on the management of pregnancy were also influenced by their female relatives' beliefs in the traditional management of pregnancy. It was therefore not surprising that advice on health and diet and the role of ceremonial rituals during pregnancy were areas where conflict sometimes became apparent.

## Annotated bibliography

Schott, J. and Henley, A. (1996) *Culture, Religion and Childbearing in a Multiracial Society: A Handbook for Health Professionals*, Oxford: Butterworth-Heinemann.
This book is mainly aimed at health care professionals to provide them with information about how to respond to the maternity care needs of ethnic minority women. The discussion includes useful background information about cultural and religious beliefs and practices surrounding pregnancy, childbirth and bereavement.

Raja, V. (1993) Conceptions of health and health care among two generations of Gujarati-speaking Hindu women in Leicester. Unpublished MPhil Thesis, Department of Sociology, University of Leicester.
The main focus of this thesis is on the concept of health and illness among Gujarati-speaking Hindu women. The author's exploration of ideas about health and illness includes beliefs about both malevolent and benevolent supernatural forces, the importance of rituals in pregnancy and beliefs about dietary prescriptions and proscriptions in pregnancy.

# 5

# Preparation for birth and childbirth experiences

The discussion in this chapter focuses on the follow-up interviews with the Gujarati and Bangladeshi Muslim women who were first interviewed in the third trimester of pregnancy. The chapter is divided into two parts. The first section discusses the women's accounts of the aspects of preparation made for childbirth; the second describes their actual experiences of childbirth in hospital. The relationship between the decisions women made in the third trimester of pregnancy and in labour and delivery are compared to explore the extent to which the women were able to determine how their labour and delivery were managed and whether there were any significant differences between the childbirth experiences of Bangladeshi and Gujarati women.

## Antenatal preparation for childbirth

From the beginning of this century, the medical management of childbirth in Britain was envisaged in broad terms, not only focusing on medical antenatal care but also on the need for the education of mothers in the art of motherhood (Oakley 1984). This approach to antenatal care was based on the assumption that lack of education was one of the factors responsible for the poor outcome of pregnancy. Oakley (1984), in a historical analysis of medical care of pregnant women, suggests that this concern was misguided in the absence of any real evidence of the efficacy of antenatal education. She also suggests that the promotion of antenatal education or parentcraft classes was based on ulterior motives, i.e. gaining control over women. Tew (1990) draws similar conclusions:

> The opportunity is taken, particularly in hospital classes, to familiarise the women with the intranatal interventions which they are likely to encounter, and to allay apprehension of the hospital settings, with its connotations of illness and emergency, the impersonality of

> its technological equipment and its sterile bustle. Thus the hospital antenatal class presents an unrivalled opportunity for putting across obstetric propaganda from authoritative sources to the target population, the women most immediately concerned, most likely to be influenced and most likely to ask for the evidence which would justify the propaganda.
>
> (Tew 1990: 93)

While an increasing number of women, including women from lower social classes, are taking advantage of antenatal classes, various randomized controlled studies have reported that, with the exception of the reduction in the use of pain-relieving drugs in labour, there is very little conclusive evidence to suggest that antenatal education is beneficial *per se* (Simkin and Enkin 1989; Tew 1990). Not only is there no conclusive evidence of the effectiveness of antenatal classes, but there is also concern about other possible adverse or harmful effects of participating in the classes:

> The extent to which fear is created rather than alleviated by classes, and whether women succumb to peer or educator pressure to conform, or refuse needed medication or intervention is completely unknown. There has been little systematic evaluation of the extent to which negative feelings of anger, guilt or inadequacy are engendered when a women's or her partner's expectations, possibly raised by the antenatal classes, are not met.
>
> (Simkin and Enkin 1989: 26)

One of the main criticisms of antenatal education, both in the past and today, is that it fails to take into account the social and economic realities of women's lives. Despite the lack of evidence to support a causal link between poor uptake of antenatal care and maternity outcome, the state and the medical profession have spared no effort in exhorting women to avail themselves of the total antenatal care package. South Asian women have been important targets of initiatives to increase compliance (see, for instance, Asian Mother and Baby Campaign; Rocheron 1988; Rocheron and Dickinson 1990).

Other perceived weaknesses of antenatal care include the different social class of the person who instructs mothers about 'mothercraft', the integration of antenatal education with medical antenatal care and the assumption that support to expectant mothers did not exist in any shape or form until the medical profession invented it. There is, however, little acknowledgement of the community-based informal support and advice which women gave and continue to give each other. As discussion in Chapter 4, page 53 suggests, in Britain there is evidence not only of a traditional form of antenatal care within the Gujarati and Bangladeshi communities, but also that older experienced women take their role of supervising and supporting younger women very seriously. Dobson (1988) also reports that the South Asian women in her study relied on female relatives and friends for advice and support in pregnancy.

There is, in fact, a growing body of literature on antenatal preparation and specifically on the rate of uptake of antenatal or parentcraft classes by women in the South Asian communities (see, for instance, McEnery and Rao 1986; Dobson 1988; Woollett *et al.* 1995; Sen and Holmes 1996). These studies point to low uptake of antenatal classes by the women within the South Asian communities. Although Woollett *et al.* (1995) report that more South Asian women in their study had attended classes than in some of the earlier studies (Homans 1982; Dobson 1988), it would seem that factors such as fluency in English and being relatively new to this country remain major barriers to the uptake of classes.

### *Attendance at parentcraft classes*

All pregnant women are expected to avail themselves of clinical antenatal care and the antenatal education provided by the NHS maternity services. Antenatal education is offered in the form of preparation classes in the community as well as in the hospital. In addition to the classes offered by the local health services, women also have the choice of attending private fee-paying classes offered by organizations such as the National Childbirth Trust and the Active Birth Movement.

The aim of antenatal preparation classes is to instruct pregnant women on the importance of health in pregnancy i.e. a healthy diet, exercise and relaxation and the harmful effects of drinking and smoking. The expectant mothers are also taught about the mechanics of labour, the use of pain-killing drugs to cope with labour pains, and medical interventions which may be performed to ensure a safe delivery. Other topics covered during classes are the care of a new baby including methods of feeding, as well as the recovery of parturient mothers in the postnatal period.

In recent years pregnant women have began to question the decisions made on their behalf in the management of their pregnancy and childbirth. Many women believe that one way to regain some control over childbirth is to acquire information from antenatal classes about the range of procedures that they might encounter so that they can make informed decisions during every stage of labour and birth.

Relatively little attention has been paid, however, to the perceptions of minority women regarding antenatal education. The discussion which follows will attempt to remedy this dearth of information by examining the uptake by the Gujarati and Bangladeshi women of parentcraft classes offered by the maternity services. The discussion will also focus on the relationship between attendance at the classes and attitudes of the women towards childbirth. The accounts of women's experiences of medical care suggest that the acceptability and accessibility of medical antenatal care were major issues for the women. The extent to which these issues influenced their participation in antenatal preparation is also explored, as is the extent to which other sources of information were available.

Many Gujarati and Bangladeshi women reported that they had received invitations to attend parentcraft or antenatal classes as a part of the antenatal care package. They were either invited to attend the classes at the hospital or arrangements were made for them to attend local community clinics. Since attendance at these classes was voluntary, women were encouraged to register their interest in them. The first interview, which took place in the third trimester of pregnancy, revealed some interesting patterns. The most marked difference was that very many more Gujarati than Bangladeshi women, both primipara (first pregnancy) and multipara, claimed that they had received an invitation to attend; because so few Bangladeshi women had received invitations, only a small number, mostly those expecting their first baby, had attended one or two classes. This contrasted sharply with the Gujarati mothers, most of whom claimed that they had attended the full course. However, there were less marked differences between Gujarati and Bangladeshi women who had been pregnant before, with only a small number from both groups reporting that they had attended one or two classes. The majority had not attended any classes; similar findings have also been reported by other studies (Dobson 1988; Leeds FHSA 1992; Woollett *et al.* 1995).

The women indicated that there were several reasons for the poor uptake and low attendance rates. Some of the most common reasons were linked to the lack of awareness of the existence or the purpose of the classes and also to whether they had received an invitation to attend. Other factors which influenced the uptake of classes were related to the women's previous experiences of participating in the classes and the benefits gained, the ease of access to classes and the extent to which women from different social and cultural backgrounds felt the need for formal preparation for childbirth.

Lack of knowledge of parentcraft classes was cited as one of the most common reasons by the Bangladeshi women for not attending parentcraft classes: 'I didn't go to any classes. I have no knowledge of where these classes are held . . . no one told me about them' (Bangladeshi mother, first pregnancy). In contrast, the majority of the Gujarati women, particularly those expecting their first baby, seemed most keen to take up the invitation to attend the classes. Their level of eagerness was evident from the fact that none of the primipara Gujarati women had missed classes and many stated that they had found them useful:

> Yes, very helpful indeed. I found it helpful to share ideas and information with other women . . . I found the information about the process of labour and the pros and cons of coping with labour pains very interesting. I feel a lot more confident as a result of attending the parentcraft classes.
>
> (Gujarati mother, first pregnancy)

A review of literature suggests that the notion of formal preparation for birth is a relatively new concept even in the western industrialized societies (Oakley 1984). In most other societies, knowledge about childbirth is acquired by assisting other women or through personal experience rather than through classes (Jeffery *et al.* 1989). The accounts of Bangladeshi women suggest that doubts about the relevance and appropriateness of classes were major barriers. For example, of the small number who had accepted the invitation to classes, only one completed the full course and the rest stopped after one or two sessions because they found the content and the method of preparing women for childbirth very embarrassing:

> The lady in the class was talking about how a baby will be delivered in hospital. I felt very embarrassed because in Bangladesh we do not talk about such things. I had gone to the parentcraft classes because I thought I had to go . . . I didn't know what it was all about but after I found out I did not want to go any more.
>
> (Bangladeshi mother, first pregnancy)

Another Bangladeshi mother who questioned the value of antenatal preparation classes echoed similar views:

> I haven't attended any classes . . . Four of my children were born in Bangladesh and the last one was born in this country. I did not attend any classes in Bangladesh or in this country. Besides I haven't got enough time to attend and moreover I think it is not necessary.
>
> (Bangladeshi mother, sixth pregnancy)

While some Bangladeshi women were offended by the explicit and detailed description of the birthing process (see also Schott and Henley 1996), this was rarely cited as a reason for non-attendance by the Gujarati women. However, few multipara Gujarati women repeated the classes in their subsequent pregnancies: some believed that it was unnecessary, as they knew all there was to know, and others felt that they had not found them useful in previous pregnancies.

Access to clinical antenatal care also contributed to the poor uptake of classes. For example, many Bangladeshi women reported that they had been invited to attend parentcraft classes run by a Bangladeshi interpreter but some were unable to go because of the lack of time, some had no-one to look after their other children, some had transport problems and the rest needed to be accompanied by their husbands: 'The Bangladeshi lady [interpreter] who works at the hospital told me about the classes for pregnant women. I haven't been able to go . . . I am afraid to go alone' (Bangladeshi mother, first pregnancy).

In recent years husbands have become increasingly involved in childbirth and there is a general expectation that they should attend classes with their wives. However, not all cultures welcome the involvement of husbands or men in childbirth. When evening classes were arranged for the benefit of women and husbands who were unable to attend daytime classes, it sometimes created problems, either because women were afraid to go out alone at night or because husbands were not willing to attend with them:

> I have never been to any classes because my husband would have had to take me to the classes. They also expect husbands to attend but my husband was not too keen to go. My husband is too busy with our family business to find time in the evening to take me to the classes.
>
> (Gujarati mother, second pregnancy)

For the majority of the Bangladeshi women, antenatal preparation was just as much an issue as the medical confirmation of pregnancy and antenatal care described in the previous chapter. While they accepted antenatal care as a prerequisite for hospital delivery, acceptance of antenatal preparation for childbirth was difficult for a number of reasons. For some, antenatal preparation was unacceptable on ideological grounds, that is, for these women childbirth was a natural event and therefore formal preparation was not considered necessary; for others access and language barriers made it difficult to participate in the classes (Thomas and Avery 1997).

The opposite seemed to be the case for the majority of the Gujarati women for whom the acceptance of neither antenatal preparation nor antenatal care seemed to be major issues. Familiarity with the western medical system certainly seemed to influence their positive attitudes towards antenatal preparation. However, while most Gujarati women accepted the concept of antenatal preparation for themselves, the involvement of husbands was less popular because of the belief that men should not be expected to play an active role during childbirth. In fact some women were reluctant to attend evening classes specifically arranged for the benefit of their husbands. If preparation for childbirth is to become more generally acceptable by women from other cultures, it is important that antenatal education should reflect the diversity of the women who attend. If, for instance, the structure and content of the course reflect only the Eurocentric view, women from other cultures may be discouraged from making use of the preparation classes to gain support through sharing and learning from each other.

An important issue which emerges from studies of this general area is that women from lower socio-economic classes were the least likely to attend antenatal classes. This is particularly significant for women in this study, many of whom were disadvantaged because of their race and socio-economic status.

### *Information about childbirth from other sources*

Traditionally in all cultures, pregnant women's knowledge about childbirth comes from the experiences of other women. This is often the only source of information available to first-time mothers. In many non-industrialized societies women also have an opportunity to gain first-hand experience by assisting other women in labour (Inch 1982; Abdulla and Zeidenstein 1982; Jeffery *et al.* 1989). In Britain, pregnant women have additional sources of information on childbirth provided by books and magazines and television and radio programmes. A large amount of health promotion literature on pregnancy and childbirth is produced by the Health Education Authority and translated into various minority ethnic languages, including Asian languages. However, there has been a great deal of concern that this literature is often not only inappropriate and insensitive, but tends to concentrate on selective health issues based on the assumptions and misconceptions of the health professionals (Bhopal and White 1993). In addition, there is considerable doubt as to whether the promotion of health through health promotion literature and mass media campaigns is the most effective and efficient method of educating the public about the prevention of ill health:

> There is a disturbing tendency in health education to regard mass media as a panacea to be applied as the treatment of choice despite the existence of convincing evidence that their effectiveness is limited.
> (Tones 1981: 98)

From the discussion above, it is evident that the uptake of antenatal preparation classes was particularly low among the Bangladeshi women. Since such classes are the main source of information about the management of childbirth in a British hospital, women who did not attend classes had to rely on other sources of formal information. However, access to sources such as printed literature, radio and television was fairly limited in the case of Bangladeshi women. Many reported that they were unable to follow television programmes and that they could not read the printed literature in English; some who had not received education beyond primary school also had difficulties reading literature in Bengali. The lack of information was particularly significant for many first-time mothers and mothers who were having their first baby in a British hospital, as they were ill-prepared to cope with a high-tech birth: 'I have not talked to anyone. I find it embarrassing. Television programmes I don't understand. Most of the things are strange to me' (Bangladeshi mother, first pregnancy).

However, as some Bangladeshi women were interviewed in the presence of their female relatives, it was difficult to gauge how much they actually knew about childbirth. It is possible that some were reluctant to acknowledge what they knew about childbirth so as not to offend the sensibilities of their relatives. For example, it was apparent that women who had personal experience of childbirth and those who had assisted other women in labour in Bangladesh were more knowledgeable. In Bangladesh their experience would have provided them with useful information to prepare for home births, assisted by lay but experienced female relatives or neighbours, but such experience would not have the same value in relation to technology-orientated hospital births.

In contrast, the majority of Gujarati women were literate in English and Gujarati and therefore were better placed to augment their existing knowledge of childbirth with information from a wide range of sources. Many women claimed that they were pleased to find the information on pregnancy and childbirth in leaflets and booklets but some believed that the information did not satisfy their needs: 'I have read all the leaflets and the booklet, which I was given at the hospital. I would like to know more about birth but the booklet does not cover it sufficiently in depth' (Gujarati mother, second pregnancy).

Some women found that the hospital booklet did not give enough detail about different methods of pain relief. This lack of information sometimes made them very anxious about whether or not they should accept drugs in labour: 'I read about pain relief in the hospital booklet, which I was given at the clinic. I did not understand everything. I find that everyone tells you different things and when I read about it I got more confused and worried' (Gujarati mother, third pregnancy).

The Gujarati women were also in the more fortunate position of being able to access information from informal sources as they were from a more established community. In contrast, it emerged that many Bangladeshi women had recently joined their husbands to settle in this country and, consequently, were isolated from social networks. For women in this position, it was a matter of chance if they obtained information from other Bangladeshi women:

> I have been talking to my neighbour who shares bed and breakfast accommodation with us. She had a baby born in this country – sometimes I ask her about the system of labour in this country. I haven't read any books or magazines or spoken to midwives because of language problems.
>
> (Bangladeshi mother, seventh pregnancy)

In the case of many Bangladeshi women it is difficult to tell whether the information they had obtained from friends and neighbours was useful as the lack of information from any other sources meant that they had no point of comparison. In addition, in a small number of cases, interviews took place in the presence of female relatives or friends which may have made it difficult to criticize the information given by such relatives and friends.

Gujarati women, on the other hand, were divided in their opinion about the value of talking to other women about childbirth. Just under half found the information provided by other women unsatisfactory. The benefit derived from talking to lay persons depended on who was giving the information. For instance, some Gujarati women felt that the information provided by their older female relatives, such as mothers-in-law or mothers, was based on old-fashioned ideas and was unhelpful to young mothers who are required to equip themselves for a hospital delivery. Some of these women felt it was more beneficial to talk to other women in their peer group:

> I have spoken to my mother-in-law but in their time it was so different. They were not expected to make any noise or feel any pain as such. My mother also told me that you can't cry out with pain or make noise but just get on with it. My mother-in-law had all her children at home so her idea of childbirth is completely different . . . I found it was more helpful to talk to my sister who just had a baby.
>
> (Gujarati mother, first pregnancy)

Other Gujarati women found the information based on the experience of other women confusing and insufficient to make decisions about pain relief.

Some mothers found they became more anxious after talking to other women:

> My cousin told me to be brave because it can be tough in labour. I have spoken to my mother-in-law but she tells me not to worry. My friend told me that it is going to be really tough . . . I feel there is something they are all hiding from me. I have been told that labour is a thousand times worse than period pain. It really scares me.
>
> (Gujarati mother, first pregnancy)

A small number of women felt that, far from being a source of useful information, programmes they had watched on childbirth had made them more apprehensive:

> It is frightening . . . You can't let your imagination run wild. They talk about episiotomy and things like that and you think 'my God, I will have to go through with it'. The film I saw of women in labour looked very painful. You don't know how painful it is going to be for you . . .
>
> (Gujarati mother, first pregnancy)

Although a few Bangladeshi women had watched programmes on childbirth, they did not express any opinion. However, one comment suggested that for some women to witness a woman giving birth was not at all unusual nor was it necessarily beneficial: 'I have watched it on television and I feel that it is something that happens to every woman. I don't know if it is helpful to learn from the television' (Bangladeshi mother, sixth pregnancy).

In short, many Asian women, and Bangladeshi women in particular, faced difficulties in obtaining information which was available to other British women. The findings of this chapter point to the isolation of the Bangladeshi women, particularly those who have settled very recently in Britain.

This is in marked contrast to Gujarati women who have at least a variety of sources of information. However, among these literate Gujarati women, the use of printed literature and television programmes was not as widespread as would be expected. This confirms the limitation of the mass media in health promotion both in reaching minority ethnic mothers and in reflecting the cultural diversity of the British population.

### *Perceptions of pain in labour and attitudes to pain-relieving drugs*

Just as there are wide cultural variations in the perception of health and illness (Raja 1993; Smaje 1995), there are similar differences in the way that pain is perceived, experienced and managed. This is equally true for the pain during childbirth. Inch (1982), for instance, suggests that the way in which women are socialized has a significant impact on attitudes towards the management of pain in labour. She cites the example of Navaho Indian women who use two different words for labour – one for 'labour' alone and another for 'the pain in labour' (Inch 1982: 93). In many industrialized nations including Britain, the technologically orientated practice of managing labour and delivery and the availability of analgesia have had a significant impact on the women's attitudes to and experiences of pain in labour. Women are led to believe that childbirth is necessarily painful and that the pain can be controlled by administration of analgesic drugs.

The fear of pain during childbirth was one of the commonest anxieties expressed by the women, particularly Gujarati women. Many first-time mothers in this group expressed doubts about their ability to handle the pain because they had nothing to compare it with, whereas women who had experienced a great deal of pain in a previous labour feared that that experience would be repeated all over again.

A pregnant woman theoretically has a choice of a range of analgesic drugs to relieve pain and discomfort during labour. The most commonly used drugs include entonox (inhalation anaesthesia), pethidine injection or local pain relief such as epidural anaesthesia. The use of pain-relieving drugs in labour depends on a number of factors such as women's perceptions of pain, the way labour is managed, previous experience of childbirth and of using drugs in labour, the availability of pain-relieving drugs and knowledge about their relative merits.

At the time of the first interview, all the pregnant women were asked if they had considered using pain-relieving drugs and, if so, what their choice would be. Interesting patterns of difference between the Gujarati and the Bangladeshi women emerged. With the exception of a small number of primipara women, who claimed to have no idea about pain-relieving drugs, the majority of Bangladeshi women reported that they would not use any drugs. The lack of awareness about the availability of pain relief in labour and the lack of previous experience of childbirth in Britain may account for the few vague responses. The more affirmative response given by the rest of the women could be interpreted in a number of ways. It is possible that, in some cases, attitudes towards pain relief reflected unfamiliarity with the administration of drugs in hospitals and, in other cases, the difference may lie in cultural attitudes towards pain in childbirth and in the way childbirth is traditionally managed. The documentary analysis of the obstetric history of Bangladeshi women revealed that the majority, indeed, had not used any form of pain relief in their previous labours. It is possible that some feel more confident in their ability to cope with their labour without drugs. As will also become apparent later in this chapter, other factors such as their late arrival at the hospital in advanced stages of labour may also account for attitudes towards pain relief.

In contrast almost all of the Gujarati women, regardless of parity, named a specific analgesic which they would prefer to use in labour. The fact that most of the women in this group had either attended some parentcraft classes or had information about drugs from other sources may have influenced their perception of pain and more ready acceptance of the need for pain-relieving drugs. This was most evident in the case of the Gujarati women with previous experience of childbirth who claimed that they could manage without pain-relieving drugs. However, it was also apparent that some Gujarati women, who had previous experience of using pain relief, had become more discriminating in their choice of analgesic. For example, some women who had accepted an epidural claimed that they would never use it again and would choose either gas/air or pethidine instead:

> I would never ask for an epidural again! In my last labour I couldn't cope with the contractions. I had asked for an epidural injection. But unfortunately it worked on one side of my body only. I could feel the pain on one half of my body. I was in agony. They couldn't understand why it wasn't working on me. I think, psychologically, it made the pain on one side of my body seem ten times worse. I will try gas/air this time but I am definitely not going to accept an epidural.
>
> (Gujarati mother, second pregnancy)

I will return to the issue of pain relief in labour later in this chapter when the women's accounts of the experiences of labour and delivery recorded in the follow-up interviews six weeks after childbirth will be explored to assess the extent to which their aspirations and expectations of childbirth were realized.

### *Feelings about forthcoming labour*

As the time of delivery approaches, it is not unusual for pregnant women to experience a certain amount of anxiety, particularly if expecting a first baby and unfamiliar with the management of labour in a hospital.

From the discussions in previous sections, it becomes apparent that not all of the women had opportunities to prepare for labour in a hospital. It was particularly significant that despite the fact that Bangladeshi women were less well informed about the management of childbirth in hospital, they appeared more confident about their ability to cope with childbirth compared with Gujarati women. It seems that attending classes or obtaining information from other sources did not necessarily inspire confidence in Gujarati women. Indeed, learning about the different medical procedures which they may have to undergo during labour may have increased their anxiety.

The nature of anxiety expressed by the women who were expecting their first baby was not peculiar to women in these two communities but is common to many other groups (Oakley 1979; McIntosh 1989). The fact that similar anxieties were also reported by a number of Gujarati women who had previous experiences of childbirth suggests that anxiety about childbirth does not necessarily diminish with parity or level of preparedness for birth. For example, although the Gujarati women appeared better informed about the management of childbirth in hospital, a majority, including those with previous experience of hospital delivery, expressed anxiety about their ability to cope. On the other hand, almost all multipara

Bangladeshi women, although less well informed about the management of childbirth than Gujarati women, did not express similar concerns. From the Bangladeshi women's point of view, it seemed as if their relatively limited formal knowledge of procedures available in relation to birth afforded them protection against anxiety related to birth. However, the explanation for the difference in attitudes becomes apparent when the women's previous experiences of childbirth were compared. For example, the majority of the multipara Bangladeshi women had had uncomplicated labours and deliveries. With the exception of two Bangladeshi women who had Caesarian sections, the rest had spontaneous and comparatively short labours. In contrast, Gujarati women, who were more knowledgeable about the management of childbirth in hospital, were drawn into the system, i.e. arrived in hospital in early labour, felt out of control, required pain relief, felt further out of control and had an assisted delivery. In the light of their previous experiences of childbirth it was not surprising that they were feeling anxious about their forthcoming childbirth. Gujarati women's accounts also suggest that merely possessing information about the management of childbirth in a hospital was not enough unless they were able to act on information and take control.

Although Gujarati women appeared to be better prepared for childbirth in a western context, this preparation did not help to reduce their anxiety. Those in their second and third pregnancy also expressed anxiety because they were afraid of having another unpleasant experience. While they were a step ahead of Bangladeshi women in terms of access to information about the management of childbirth they were not able to use this information to their advantage.

Bangladeshi women on the whole appeared to be less anxious and, in fact, those who had previous home births in Bangladesh felt more confident because they were under the impression that delivery in a hospital is a lot easier and safer. In addition, women whose previous experiences of childbirth were straightforward did not express any anxiety. Bangladeshi women expecting their first babies also felt confident in their ability to cope with labour because many were not aware of medical procedures or interventions which may have caused anxiety.

## Experiences of childbirth

### *Introduction*

In the west, medicalization and almost 100 per cent hospitalization has divorced childbirth from its traditional social context. This has fostered an impression that childbirth is an illness and the only proper place for its treatment is the hospital under the supervision of medical experts, rather than the home or other community settings. It is widely argued that hospitals, which are well equipped with modern technology, are far safer places for delivery and also that the hospitalization of childbirth has contributed to the reduction in maternal and child mortality. However, neither of these claims has been supported by evidence (Oakley 1984; Tew 1990).

Implicit in the medicalization of childbirth is the assumption that pregnancy and childbirth are potentially abnormal and hence medical intervention is fully justified in all cases. While technological innovations have their roots in science, there is mounting concern that many new techniques have been introduced without any clear evidence of either their effectiveness in improving outcomes or the long-term safety of some procedures. For example, a range of innovations such as induction, ultrasound, foetal monitoring and biochemical placental function tests are routinely used without paying due consideration to the possibility of long-term danger (Inch 1982; Reid 1990).

Historically and cross-culturally, the management of childbirth was predominantly located in the hands of women (Versluysen 1981; Inch 1982). While women have gradually lost control over the management of childbirth in western industrialized countries (Robinson 1990), this process of transformation has not taken place to the same degree in non-industrialized countries. For instance, in many parts of the Indian subcontinent, particularly in the rural areas, childbirth is still managed by untrained but experienced women, and men only play a marginal role. A study by Patricia Jeffery and her colleagues (1989) of Hindu and Muslim women in rural north India highlights the central role of female relatives and traditional birth attendants. Blanchet (1984) provides a further example of female-centred management of childbirth in Bangladesh. In addition, even in Britain, older Asian women play an important role in the management of pregnancy and childbirth, as Homans's (1980) comparative study of British and Asian women's experiences of pregnancy and childbirth shows.

The existence of a strong tradition of female-centred reproductive care in the Indian subcontinent has a particular significance to British Asian women for a variety of reasons. For example, many Bangladeshi women having their babies in Britain have recently migrated from Bangladesh and therefore have fresh memories of reproductive care controlled by female relatives and traditional birth attendants. Similarly, although a majority of the Gujarati women were born in East Africa and were more familiar with the western model of childbirth, older female relatives to a large extent influenced their behaviour during childbirth.

### *Gujarati and Bangladeshi women's experiences of childbirth in hospital*

Although childbirth is a natural physiological process, for the individual woman it is a unique experience. On the emotional level every woman has a different response to each birth, so that one birth may be remembered as a painful and distressing experience while another may be remembered as a relatively easy and pleasant experience. The way women respond is partly emotional and partly cultural. The physical aspects of childbirth are also culturally defined so that, although women from different cultures go through the same physiological process, each culture attaches different values and meanings to this process (Kitzinger 1978; MacCormack 1982). Consequently women from other cultures who have recently settled in Britain face great tension in trying to relate their childbirth experiences in the new setting to their own cultural context.

In some respects the experiences of childbirth of Asian women are not very different from those of other British women. However, in order to understand the way Gujarati and Bangladeshi women perceive their childbirth experiences in Britain, it is necessary to set their experiences within the context of the management of childbirth in the country of origin.

The majority of Bangladeshi women in the study had come from the rural district of Sylhet, in Bangladesh, where home births were normal and women only went into local hospitals if complications developed during pregnancy. More than half the Bangladeshi women interviewed had given birth at home in their previous pregnancies and some of these were contemplating their first experience of giving birth in a hospital. The following interview conducted with a key informant within the Bangladeshi community provides a typical example of a home birth:

> When a woman starts her labour she remains active doing her tasks until she is in the last stages of labour. At this stage she will go into a partitioned room where she will be attended to by one or two female relatives who are used to helping in childbirth. Her female relatives would give her support and encouragement throughout the labour until the baby is born. If labour is difficult the mother or mother-in-law would send for a village midwife or *dai* who uses her manipulation skills to speed up a protracted labour. If labour is difficult the mother is given a drink of water containing a rare dried flower to hasten the labour.
>
> (Bangladeshi Community Social Worker)

In contrast, the majority of the Gujarati women were from East Africa where home births had been phased out in favour of maternity homes or hospitals. Their knowledge of home births was therefore based on the experiences of their mothers and mothers-in-law. The following is a generalized description of childbirth in a British hospital, with which these women were more familiar.

Before the end of pregnancy a woman is given instructions to report the onset of her labour. When the labour starts a woman leaves the familiarity of her home to go into hospital where she is looked after by a team of obstetric staff who are at the same time looking after other women in labour. Unless a woman has a labour companion she may be left alone while the staff are attending to other women. If on arrival at the hospital her labour is making slow progress, it may be accelerated with the rupture of the membranes or by use of a hormone preparation. If a woman finds her labour too painful she is offered pain-relieving drugs. If at this stage a woman is unable to deliver her baby, further medical intervention follows in the form of forceps, episiotomy or Caesarean section. Inch (1982: 36) coined the phrase 'cascade of intervention' to describe how medical intervention in the early stages of labour leads to a situation where further medical intervention becomes unavoidable.

In the past few years, pregnant women and organizations fighting for the rights of women to have more control during childbirth have questioned the increasing use of modern technology in the hospital (Oakley 1984). As the discussion at the beginning of this chapter suggests, women who have very little information about the management of childbirth in a hospital have a limited range of information on which to base their decisions. However, as will become clear later, being well informed is only a part of the struggle in avoiding unnecessary medical interference; the other challenge is to be assertive when confronted with expert medical advice.

### *Women's experiences of hospital delivery*

Pregnant women are advised to contact the hospital labour ward when they notice the first signs of labour, i.e. strong contractions coming at short intervals or the breaking of the bag of waters surrounding the baby. The labour ward staff make the decision about the time of admission. A hospital delivery makes it necessary for a woman in labour to leave her home environment and make a journey to the hospital. This causes added anxiety to pregnant women and their partners who are worried about getting there in time.

On the other hand, women who do not see their labour in terms of distinct stages may not feel it necessary to rush into hospital until the baby is ready to be born. It became apparent from the accounts of some Bangladeshi women that the decision about how soon the hospital should be notified after the labour has started seemed to be guided by the practice in Bangladesh, where women in labour continue with their normal activities until it is nearly time to deliver the baby.

The timing of admission into hospital was an important factor in determining the management of the childbirth and the outcome of the pregnancy. For instance, it is just as vital for a woman not to delay her admission if she has any abnormal symptoms as it is for her not to be admitted too early in labour. The accounts of Gujarati and Bangladeshi women revealed that, for those who had gone into labour spontaneously, there was a significant difference in the time of notifying the hospital about their condition and their arrival at the hospital.

Many Gujarati women, including women with previous experience of labour, had arrived at the hospital in early labour soon after contacting the labour ward. The interviews with Gujarati women revealed that a majority had contacted the local hospital as soon as they noticed the first signs of labour and had not lost any time in arriving at the hospital. There were several reasons to account for this pattern of behaviour. For example, the level of eagerness for early admission into hospital was partly related to their anxiety but also to their perceptions of hospital as a place of safety. This was understandable as none of them had considered or had any previous experience of home delivery. In addition, many Gujarati women had attended antenatal classes and had more access to information on the management of childbirth in a hospital. Therefore, they were responding to the instructions they had received about the need to report the onset of their labour. A Gujarati mother who was advised to wait at home until her labour was well established found it difficult to understand why she was not admitted sooner:

> My labour started with a backache and I also had a 'show' [expulsion of mucous plug from the cervix]. When I telephoned the hospital they told me to wait until the contractions were coming every ten minutes. In the meantime they advised me to take paracetamol for the backache. This went on for three days and each time I was told to wait until the contractions started or if my waters went. On the third day I insisted that I must have a check up with a monitor to see if I was in labour and only then they admitted me.
>
> (Gujarati mother, first pregnancy)

The reactions of the Bangladeshi women were very different. With two exceptions, both expecting their first baby, the women had arrived at hospital in the advanced stages of labour. It would appear that Bangladeshi women were anxious to delay their admission to hospital for several reasons. Apart from their views on the traditional management of labour, many Bangladeshi women had to rely on their husbands for support, for making contact with the hospital and for arranging transportation. Although Bangladeshi women on the whole accepted hospital delivery, they were also anxious to spend as little time as possible in an alien environment where they would have difficulty in communicating with the hospital staff. In addition, many women without extended family support had to take into consideration the welfare of their other children:

> My labour pains started at lunchtime. My husband called the ambulance at 11 o'clock at night when my pains were too much for me. I didn't want to go to hospital too soon . . . I have to think about my three daughters. For my husband it would be too much . . . the eldest is only six years. I do not know many people here who could look after my children. I am also afraid to go to hospital without my husband because I do not understand English.
>
> (Bangladeshi mother, fifth pregnancy)

Bangladeshi women with previous experience of childbirth also seemed to be using their own judgement as to when it was the right time to go into hospital. Their comments suggest that they were more attuned to their bodies and did not see the need to rush into hospital with the first twinge: 'My pain started three days before the actual delivery. My husband called an ambulance at about 10 p.m. on the 6th of October and I had my baby at 4 a.m. My labour lasted four to five hours' (Bangladeshi mother, sixth pregnancy).

The practice of delaying admission to the maternity hospital appears to be widespread. A Bengali interpreter who was one of the key informants in the study reported that many women were afraid of medical intervention:

> Some women wait at home until the labour is well advanced and sometimes women are admitted just in time for the delivery. Some of these women have heard stories from other women that if they arrive too early in labour then they would have a Caesarean section. In my experience, I found that quite a few didn't come into hospital until they were in full labour. Some people also believe, especially some husbands, that the doctor may carry out a sterilization while a woman is having a Caesarean.
>
> (Bangladeshi Hospital Interpreter)

Schott and Henley (1996: 149) argue that some ethnic minority women's experiences of poor care or inappropriate treatment or being subjected to racist abuse and rudeness induce fear and distrust of health professionals. In these circumstances it is understandable that they may wish to restrict their contact with health professionals to an absolute minimum.

In the case of the women whose labours had started spontaneously, it was evident that the timing of arrival at hospital had a direct impact on how their labour and delivery were managed. For instance, the Bangladeshi women who had delayed their arrival reported that they had delivered their babies soon after they were admitted into the labour ward and the majority had a normal delivery without medical intervention. The claims made by the women were confirmed by their obstetric records. In contrast, the Gujarati women who had arrived at the hospital in the early stages of labour had experiences which mirrored Inch's (1982) 'cascade of intervention'. They reported that, after they were admitted into the labour ward, they felt totally out of control because their labours were accelerated with hormone preparations and the only way they could bear the pain was to accept pain-relieving drugs:

> When I arrived at the hospital they told me that I was in early labour. I was in a lot of pain. I was given pethidine, which didn't help much. They gave me epidural and in between I was using a gas mask. I then stopped dilating so they set up a hormone drip. The third top-up of epidural only worked on one side and I started to feel sick. When it came to pushing, I couldn't push because I felt numb from waist down . . . The baby started to show signs of distress . . . In the end I had a forceps delivery with episiotomy as well as bad tear. I was very upset and angry . . . the midwife was supposed to encourage me to push the baby; instead I was left to get on and that is why the baby was in distress.
>
> (Gujarati mother, first pregnancy)

Other Gujarati women who had arrived at the hospital in early labour had similar experiences because they were unable to control what was happening to them or to challenge the decisions made by the obstetric staff:

> I did not have any contractions or any pain. My labour was accelerated with a hormone drip. I was also given an injection of epidural in my back at the same time. The midwife told me that I wouldn't be able to cope without painkillers because I was induced. I had not asked for the epidural but I thought the midwife knew what was good for me. After I was in labour for over twelve hours they decided to do a Caesarean because the baby was upside down. They had not realized that the baby was coming down feet first although I had told them that I could feel the baby's head on the side of my ribs. They wouldn't believe me and said 'Mrs P don't worry, everything is just fine. We know what we are doing.' In the end it was too late to do a Caesarean and I delivered him feet first. I had forceps delivery and needed a lot of stitches.
>
> (Gujarati mother, second pregnancy)

### *Women's experience of induction*

As the time for the delivery draws near, most women feel a certain amount of impatience. One of the major factors which contributes to this impatience is the importance attached to the estimated or expected date of delivery. The medical management of labour not only places greater emphasis on the division of labour into distinct stages but also places a time limit on how long each stage is allowed to proceed unaided, although there is often insufficient evidence to justify interventions (Enkin *et al.* 1990). If the progress at any stage is deemed to be slow, the process is speeded up with an artificial stimulation of labour and, in some cases, with a Caesarean section. In countries such as Bangladesh, where maternity services are not developed on the same scale as in the industrialized countries, pregnant women wait for nature to take its course and are not dictated to by expected dates of delivery or notions of different stages of labour (Blanchet 1984; Jeffery *et al.* 1989).

Although there may be pressing medical reasons for bringing forward the date of delivery by artificial means, the practice of induction two weeks past the expected date of delivery often causes concern to women who would prefer to start labour spontaneously. A majority of women if left alone start labour between the 38th and 42nd week of pregnancy as was the case with over a third of the Gujarati and Bangladeshi women. For instance, with the exception of two Bangladeshi women who had elective Caesarean, the rest had gone into labour spontaneously with either the rupture of membranes or with the regular contractions of the womb. A similar pattern of spontaneous labour was reported by a majority of Gujarati women, with the exception of a small number of women who had their pregnancy artificially induced because they were overdue by ten days. Gujarati women whose labours were induced were upset by the fact that they were not allowed time for their labour to start naturally. One Gujarati woman claimed that she was made to feel guilty for resisting induction:

> At the end of my pregnancy I was feeling fine, had no problems. At my last appointment, in the week when the baby was due, the doctor talked about induction. I was scared – worried about the baby. After my labour was induced, I had accepted epidural as I could not cope with the pain and the baby started to show signs of distress. After the baby was born, the doctor made me feel even worse by saying that it was just as well things worked out otherwise I would have ended up with a section. He finished by telling me that I should always listen to their advice, they [doctors] don't say things for fun.
>
> (Gujarati mother, first pregnancy)

Another Gujarati mother with a similar experience of induction felt that the treatment she had received was insensitive and had made her feel very anxious about going into hospital again:

> I was overdue but I did not want to be induced because it didn't feel right. They didn't explain what was going on after I was induced. I was in pain for twenty-four hours before I was taken down to the delivery room. I was screaming and crying all the time. I didn't have anyone to comfort me. I also had the drip inserted in wrong place by a midwife and she even told me what she had done! I couldn't believe that it could be possible to be treated like that . . .
>
> (Gujarati mother, second pregnancy)

Gujarati women's concerns about induction were similar to those expressed by many white women (cf Cartwright 1977; McIntosh 1989).

It would seem that Bangladeshi women who had elective Caesarean sections were just as unhappy about medical intervention. One of these mothers reported that she had resisted her admission into hospital until a few hours before her operation:

> The doctor at the hospital wanted to admit me a day before the operation. I was not very happy about the operation. I wanted to stay at home as long as possible in case my pains started. Unfortunately the pains did not start as I hoped they might do in the night. I went to the hospital in the morning and in the afternoon I had my operation.
>
> (Bangladeshi mother, second pregnancy)

To sum up then, the accounts of the birth experiences of the Gujarati women suggest that not only were they open to the idea of hospital delivery but that they also sought the security provided by medical experts by arriving at the hospital as soon as they suspected the first signs of labour. The behaviour of many women, particularly Gujarati women who had received instructions about the appropriate time to report the onset of labour, was not unusual as they were, after all, only following the instructions they had been given.

In contrast, the behaviour of many Bangladeshi women, including those expecting their first baby, suggested that the decision to delay their admission into the hospital was based on their own instincts although, in some cases, women had other pressing reasons to delay admission. While Gujarati women sometimes became caught up within the hospital system and became passive recipients of care, the Bangladeshi women, intentionally or unintentionally, avoided getting caught up in the system by delaying their arrival at the hospital. Consequently they were less disappointed with their experiences.

### *Women's experiences of pain relief in labour*

It was evident in the discussion above that there were considerable differences between Gujarati and Bangladeshi women in their knowledge, attitudes and choice of pain relief. The women's accounts of childbirth in the follow-up interviews were analysed to see if there were significant differences in the use of pain relief between those who had made a prior decision about pain relief and those who had not and if their attitudes had changed in the light of their experiences.

When the women's accounts about pain relief before and after childbirth were compared, an interesting pattern emerged. For example, a majority of Bangladeshi women, who were either undecided or did not think pain-relieving drugs were necessary, claimed that they had managed to cope without any pain relief. The only exceptions were three women who had a general anaesthetic for Caesarean sections. On the other hand, with one exception, all the Gujarati women had used at least one form of analgesic drugs and in some cases two or more.

From earlier discussions concerning admission into hospital it would appear that the time of arrival and the progress of labour might also have determined whether or not pain-relieving drugs were necessary. For instance, a number of the Bangladeshi women claimed that, although they had been in labour for some hours, they had not called for an ambulance until they were nearly ready to deliver. It was evident that some had delayed calling an ambulance for a variety of personal and practical reasons. However, the fact that they had arrived at the hospital in the final stages of labour, having completed the earlier stages in the familiar surroundings of their homes, may have removed the need for pain relief.

Yet, though many Bangladeshi women claimed that they had not used any pain-relieving drugs in their labours, documentary analysis of their hospital medical records revealed that for a small number this had not been the case. This anomaly suggests that these women, none of whom had any previous experience of delivery in a hospital, had accepted pain-relieving drugs without their knowledge or consent. Moreover, the following comments show that many Bangladeshi women were confused about the administration of drugs in labour: 'When I was admitted into the hospital, the baby was ready to be born. The doctor gave me an injection as I was in too much pain trying to push the baby out. I do not know the name of the medicine I was given' (Bangladeshi mother, sixth pregnancy).

The fact that the injection of syntometrine, which is routinely administered to speed up the involution of the womb, was often mistaken for pain-relieving drugs by some women suggests that little effort was made to share relevant information with women. This broadly confirms the findings of Fleissig's (1993) study. Another Bangladeshi mother, whose medical record showed that she had not been given any pain-relieving drugs, also believed that she had accepted pain-relieving drugs when she was given a routine injection of syntometrine: 'I was taken to the hospital when it was time for the baby to be born. In the hospital I was given some liquid medicine through my arm as I was very weak and could not push the baby. I also had another injection to make it less painful to push' (Bangladeshi mother, seventh pregnancy).

The more widespread use of drugs among Gujarati women may be linked to the timing of their admission in hospital and how far advanced they were in labour. It is also possible that the hospital environment and the length of time spent in the labour ward may have added to the stress of labour and may have increased their need for pain relief.

However, it was also evident that knowledge about availability had made it easier for Gujarati women to ask for pain-relieving drugs. The women's accounts highlighted further differences among the Gujarati women who had made a prior decision about the choice of pain-relieving drugs. For instance, with the exception of two Gujarati women, they all used their preferred choice of pain-relieving drugs and about half had also used additional drugs besides the ones they had originally chosen. Although the use of drugs was related to their pain threshold and the nature of their labour, i.e. whether the labour was allowed to progress smoothly or was artificially speeded up, it seems that once the decision to use drugs was made, their use during labour became inevitable. It was particularly striking that only a small number of the Bangladeshi women claimed that they had accepted pain-relieving drugs and that their use of drugs was restricted to one type of drug. It would appear that the women who were the least knowledgeable about pain relief seemed to fare a lot better in terms of coping with their labour pains. In contrast with the Gujarati women, it would seem that Bangladeshi women, and especially those with previous experience of labour, had little expectation of drugs to provide relief.

### *Management of delivery*

It would appear that poor attendance at antenatal classes, especially among the Bangladeshi women, did not affect the outcome of pregnancy. On the contrary, with the exception of three Bangladeshi women who had Caesarean sections, babies were delivered without any medical interventions and, in most cases, without the use of pain-relieving drugs. Of the three women who had assisted deliveries, two had an elective Caesarean section on medical grounds and only one had an emergency Caesarean section.

In contrast, although a majority of the Gujarati women started labour spontaneously at home, a third from this group claimed that their labour was accelerated after admission into hospital and the remainder of Gujarati women reported that they had been admitted for elective induction. Women whose labours were induced or accelerated found that they could not cope with the intensity of contractions and required additional pain-relieving drugs. A mother who was overwhelmed by pain after her labour was accelerated remarked:

> When I arrived at the hospital I was getting mild contractions but once they set the drip up to speed up the labour the contractions became very strong and very painful. I tried the gas mask but I found it did not help so I had pethidine, which made me very drowsy. I could still feel the pain. By the time I was asked to push I felt totally out of control. I wanted someone to take the baby out.
>
> (Gujarati mother, second pregnancy)

Some of these women found that the combination of acceleration with a hormone drip and pain-relieving drugs made them feel unable to manage the last stages of labour on their own. A number of Gujarati women had an episiotomy, sometimes to facilitate forceps delivery. One particular mother who was distressed and unable to push the baby out found that she did not feel strong enough to object to the medical student making unsuccessful attempts to apply the forceps. She continued:

> The medical student had four goes at applying forceps which really upset me because it was unnecessary. I was not in a fit state to object. I think the senior doctor should have taken over when the student doctor failed to do it correctly. The forceps caused a lot of bad bruising on me and my baby. The bruising made me bedridden for three weeks.
>
> (Gujarati mother, second pregnancy)

In summarizing the women's experiences of childbirth, it seems that being well informed about the management of childbirth through antenatal classes was not enough since many were only exposed to the way childbirth was managed in hospital. Many of the medical interventions such as acceleration and episiotomy were put across as routine hospital procedures. For this reason, some Gujarati women were not able to assert themselves in the presence of medical experts. However, this problem is not unique to Gujarati women, as a similar loss of confidence by other British women, when confronted first by a painful labour and second by medical experts advocating a particular course of action, has been widely reported (Oakley 1979; Kitzinger 1987).

The more ready acceptance of medical procedures in labour made it difficult for Gujarati women to question the way their labour and delivery were managed despite the fact that a majority were fluent in English. On the other hand, the Bangladeshi women, despite the many disadvantages they experienced, managed to retain some control by delaying their arrival at the hospital.

### *Labour companion*

In recent years, one of the most significant changes in attitudes towards childbirth has been associated with the role husbands are expected to play in childbirth (Barbour 1990; Niven 1992). In Britain, many Asian men find themselves fulfilling the role of labour companion, which traditionally would be fulfilled by female members of their family.

Although the practice of having husbands present during labour is becoming more common, it still remains problematic for many South Asian couples and their families for cultural and religious reasons (Homans 1982; Currer 1986; Woollett and Dosanjh-Matwala 1990a). Almost all the Gujarati women reported that their husbands had stayed with them for the major part of their labour and delivery. In the case of the Bangladeshi women, a majority had been accompanied to the hospital by their husbands, most of whom had kept away from the labour ward unless their presence was absolutely necessary.

Hospitalization of childbirth and the greater emphasis placed on the presence of husbands during childbirth has effectively devalued the traditional supporting role of female relatives. Almost all the Gujarati women stated that they expected their husbands to be present at the birth because they believed that this was expected of them: 'It is the done thing these days . . . everyone expects that husbands should stay with their wives.' In a small number of cases, the Gujarati women reported that their female relatives had accompanied them to the hospital but had left as soon as their husbands had joined them. It was interesting to note that the female relatives who played an active role in providing support during pregnancy found that they temporarily lost their role to a male member of their family because the birth took place in the hospital. However, they were called upon to resume their role once the woman was discharged home. This often caused resentment among female relatives, especially among some mothers-in-law who felt that childbirth was women's business and their sons should not be exposed to childbirth (Woollett and Dosanjh-Matwala 1990a). Some of these conflicting issues are revisited in Chapter 7.

Turning now to the Bangladeshi women's labour companions, it appears that the role of labour companion is forced upon husbands, and many fill this role out of necessity rather than the express desire of either the childbearing women or the men themselves. Since many of the Bangladeshi women were not able to speak English, they needed their husbands to accompany them to hospital and act as their interpreters.

Separate interviews with a Bangladeshi interpreter and a Bangladeshi community social worker revealed that many Bangladeshi women felt very uncomfortable about being exposed in front of their husbands and preferred them to wait outside the labour ward. However, some Bangladeshi men considered their presence at the hospital necessary to ensure that their wives' purdah was not violated by the presence of male doctors. They often insisted that there should be nobody present in the labour room except female staff. Some Bangladeshi husbands also insisted that they should be consulted and their permission obtained before any medical procedures were carried out: 'If any pain killers are given or if any medical procedures are carried out in labour, the midwife or the doctor has to ask the permission of the husband first because a woman would not agree to anything without her husband's consent' (Bangladeshi Interpreter).

It would appear that, because of the hospitalization of childbirth, Asian men were forced into a new role which required them to make important decisions on procedures they knew very little about (Perkins 1980). The Bangladeshi men were not alone in facing this problem, as the following account of a young Gujarati mother illustrates:

> After I was admitted into the hospital, I was given sleeping pills and told to rest before induction in the morning. My husband went home and in the middle of the night I started to leak and my cramps got worse. When the midwife examined me, she couldn't find baby's heartbeat and my waters were brown. She asked me to sign a consent form for a Caesarean. My husband had told me not to sign anything. I didn't know what to do. I didn't want to disobey my husband but at the same time the midwife was pressing me to sign the forms. I was so frightened. After the midwife warned me that I was putting my baby at risk I signed the form.
>
> (Gujarati mother, first pregnancy)

### *Reactions after childbirth*

The way a woman reacts to the birth of her baby is very complex (Oakley 1979; McIntosh 1989). Immediately after birth, emotions can range from elation to a feeling of complete detachment from the reality of the event. No matter how many times a woman gives birth, her reaction is unique and unpredictable. The most common reaction expressed soon after the baby makes its appearance are relief that the hard work is finally over and that the baby is normal and healthy.

The experiences of the Gujarati and Bangladeshi women suggested that their reactions were affected by a number of factors: for instance, whether the mother was emotionally prepared to have a baby, whether the pregnancy was intended or unintended, whether there was any anxiety concerning the baby during the pregnancy. Other important issues were the way their labour and delivery were managed and whether their expectations of childbirth were realized. At the time of the first interview, the women's reactions to their pregnancy had reflected a certain amount of uncertainty about their pregnancies and some had expressed concern about the outcome, in particular the sex of the baby they were carrying.

With three exceptions, the Gujarati women were very happy with the outcome of their pregnancies. Those who had given birth to a son were particularly pleased. This was because most were in their first or second pregnancy and did not already have sons. It would also seem that the women with daughters who gave birth to a son at the end of the current pregnancy had a much more positive attitude towards their labour in retrospect, even though some of these women were initially very unhappy to find themselves pregnant:

> Although at first I was not at all pleased to be pregnant I was overjoyed and excited to know it was a boy. My mother-in-law's attitude towards me has also changed because it is a boy. If I had a girl I wouldn't have been so excited, probably I would have cried with disappointment. I was very pleased with the whole experience. I think I had a much easier labour compared to my last labour. I am still on a high having given birth to a son.
>
> (Gujarati mother, second pregnancy)

One Bangladeshi mother on the other hand was very upset because she had given birth to her fifth daughter:

> We were hoping and praying that this pregnancy I would have a son. My husband and I were disappointed because if we had a son we would not have any more babies but now we will have to try again. When the midwife told me that it was a girl, I cried – no, not another girl. I was very sad and upset at first but now I am okay.
>
> (Bangladeshi mother, fifth pregnancy)

Although women who already had a daughter or daughters were under considerable pressure to produce a son, many mothers who were expecting their first baby had also secretly wished for a son so that they would be spared the pressure in their subsequent pregnancy/ies. However, they often did not openly voice their anxiety about the sex of the baby until after the baby was born:

> We didn't know the sex of the baby until the nurse brought her back and announced it was a girl. I felt sorry for my husband because it was a girl. I didn't want to hold her or even to look at her. I didn't feel any attachment towards her. I felt bit strange towards her – I didn't want to grab her like other mothers do. My husband pointed to the similarity between myself and the baby but I was not able to respond. It took me a whole day to get used to the idea. I refused to hold her; maybe if it were a son I would have grabbed him. I thought I was carrying a son because everyone told me that it was going to be a son.
>
> (Gujarati mother, first pregnancy)

A Bangladeshi mother and a Gujarati mother who had had very painful labour experiences felt that they were far too upset after the delivery to rejoice at the birth of their babies. The Bangladeshi mother who had had an emergency Caesarean section explained: 'After the baby was born I felt that I would never get pregnant again. I found the labour very painful and then I had to have a lot of stitches afterwards. I was relieved to know that my daughter was healthy but I was not happy with my labour' (Bangladeshi mother, first pregnancy).

A number of Gujarati mothers who also had painful experiences of childbirth felt that the pain of epidural, episiotomy or forceps had left them with unpleasant memories of an experience, which they would not like to repeat.

It was clear that the ambiguous feelings of women who had either not intended to have a baby or had expressed ambiguous attitudes towards their pregnancy did not diminish immediately after the birth of their baby. For example, a Gujarati mother who was very unhappy about her unplanned pregnancy and had tried unsuccessfully to abort her baby claimed that she felt completely drained of emotion and did not even wish to acknowledge the birth of her baby:

> I would never go through it again. Never, mostly because of the pain. The last two labours were not as painful. This time the labour was short but much more unbearable. I was feeling very anxious throughout my labour. I was very upset because I was convinced that I had harmed my baby by taking so many drugs in my early pregnancy . . . I don't even remember seeing the baby born. I did not feel anything when my husband told me that we had a son. I did not feel like handling the baby until the second day when I had a good look to see if his body was deformed. I felt relieved to see he had all his toes and fingers and he was not harmed by the medicine. I am glad now that everything worked out in the end and I am pleased he is here.
>
> (Gujarati mother, third pregnancy)

Another Gujarati woman who was very unhappy about her third unplanned pregnancy continued to express negative feelings about her childbirth experience:

> I asked for pethidine because I didn't want to put up with any pain. I told the midwife she should either give me some pethidine or do a Caesarean. I was not in the mood to go through labour – I felt indifferent to what was happening to me. When he was born I was relieved that the pain was over. I felt numb – no feeling at all. Okay he is there; I will just have to get on with him.
>
> (Gujarati mother, fourth pregnancy)

Another Gujarati mother who was unhappy about her pregnancy complained that she had sacrificed her career to please her husband and his family by having a baby when she was not ready to be a mother. She felt depressed because her baby was born prematurely, and could not hide her resentment towards her in-laws who thought of her only as someone who could give them a grandson:

> Since I have brought my baby home my whole life revolves round the baby. I am not allowed to go out anywhere. It is just as well that I have produced a son; I think my life would have been made too difficult for me if it had been a daughter. My mother-in-law makes me feel that I should have no other interest other than the care of her grandson.
>
> (Gujarati mother, first pregnancy)

A young mother who was not prepared for an emergency Caesarean section felt dazed and totally out of control because her husband and the hospital staff appeared to be making all the decisions. Her dilemma was evident from the time she was asked to sign a consent form for an emergency section while her husband had explicitly forbidden her to sign any forms:

> When I came round I was in shock. For the first two days I was in so much of a daze, I never asked why I couldn't see the baby. It is strange that I didn't ask, I really don't know why. I didn't understand why she was in an incubator or know what was wrong with her. I was disappointed with the way things worked out.
>
> (Gujarati mother, first pregnancy)

With the exception of two Bangladeshi women who were unhappy that their babies were born by Caesarean section, the rest were relieved that their deliveries had ended safely. Those who accepted their pregnancies as destined by their fate appeared to accept childbirth and the birth of their babies with equanimity. Bangladeshi women with high parity seemed to be particularly undaunted by childbirth:

> I gave birth to my four children at home in Bangladesh with just my mother-in-law. I had no problems, as my labours were very quick. I am an experienced mother so I can manage my delivery but I was pleased when it was over and the baby was all right physically.
>
> (Bangladeshi mother, sixth pregnancy)

Some Bangladeshi mothers appeared to be more concerned about the health of their babies and about getting away from the hospital, where they felt ill at ease, to return to other children at home. A mother whose underweight baby was admitted to the special care unit felt very depressed because she was torn between the idea of leaving her baby in the baby unit and her need to care for her other children at home:

> My labour was not difficult. It lasted only three to four hours. My baby was born earlier than expected and only weighed about four pounds. I did not have my baby with me because he was in a baby ward. I was worried about my son because he was underweight. I was anxious to go home because of my other children . . .
>
> (Bangladeshi mother, seventh pregnancy)

## Summary

While each mother's experience of childbirth was perceived by her as a unique event, there were a number of major differences between the way Bangladeshi and Gujarati women coped with their labour and deliveries. It became apparent, for instance, that their experiences were affected by their expectations of the management of labour and that this, in turn, influenced how eager they were to be admitted into hospital.

The experiences of Gujarati women suggested that they were eager to be admitted into hospital in early labour because they were accustomed to the idea of a hospital as a safe place to give birth. In addition, the majority were also eager to obey instructions concerning admission into hospital. Consequently they tended to arrive at the hospital, as instructed, in the early stages of labour.

On the other hand, a majority of Bangladeshi women were more familiar with birth at home and as a result they did not see any reason for rushing into hospital in the early stages of labour. In addition, hospital admission created problems such as language difficulties and having to rely increasingly on their husbands for moral and physical support in labour. As a result, it was not surprising that many women delayed admission until they were in advanced labour.

The timing of admission seemed to play a crucial role in determining how their labour progressed and how it was managed. For instance, Gujarati women who arrived early found that, although they had started their labour spontaneously, once they were admitted they were not able to avoid medical intervention. Partly as a result of medical intervention and partly due to their more favourable attitude towards pain-relieving drugs, many Gujarati women found that they could not cope with labour pains. It was also interesting to note that not only were the Gujarati women more willing to entertain the idea of pain-relieving drugs during their pregnancy but that they also used additional drugs besides the ones they had originally intended. In contrast, the experiences of the majority of the Bangladeshi women suggested that, because they delayed their admission into hospital until they were in well-established labour, they were able to avoid medical intervention and also the need for pain-relieving drugs.

For the majority of the Gujarati women, the participation of husbands during labour was not a major issue, although it did not always meet with the approval of their older relatives. In contrast, for many Bangladeshi women who did not share similar views, the involvement of husbands during labour was culturally unacceptable for them and for their husbands. The experience of the Bangladeshi women highlights the difficulties encountered by women who have to manage without the traditional female support during childbirth, in addition to being confined in an alien hospital environment.

The range of feelings expressed by the women after childbirth in many ways reflected the attitudes they had adopted during their pregnancy. It would seem that the women, in particular Gujarati women who had either not planned to have a baby or had ambiguous attitudes towards their pregnancy, continued to express similarly ambivalent attitudes towards their childbirth experiences. In contrast, the Bangladeshi women, who accepted their pregnancies as ordained by the will of God, seemed also to perceive their childbirth experiences in the same light.

The women who thought that their labour and delivery were badly managed and the women who had failed to produce a male child were the most upset by their experiences. The accounts of the women's experiences give some indication of the issues which confront women from different cultural and social backgrounds when they give birth in a hospital setting.

## Annotated bibliography

There is a large volume of feminist literature on childbirth and related health issues. Although the concerns of childbearing women in the last two decades have had a significant impact on policy and practice governing maternity services, some areas of concern still remain. Very few publications listed here have examined the issues facing minority ethnic women, although the concerns they have raised also have implications for women other than white women.

Garcia, J., Kilpatrick, R. and Richards, M. (eds) (1990) *The Politics of Maternity Care: Services for Childbearing Women in Twentieth-Century Britain.* Oxford: Clarendon Press.

This collection of essays provides historical and social perspectives on recent developments in childbirth practices and discusses their impact on mothers, the professionals and pressure groups.

Oakley, A. (1984) *The Captured Womb.* Oxford: Blackwell.

This book gives an insight into the historical development of maternity care. It traces development from the eighteenth and nineteenth centuries when doctors were rarely involved in the care of pregnant women to the late twentieth century where care of pregnant women has increasingly come under the control of male doctors. Ann Oakley discusses the impact of medicalization of motherhood and the struggles women have faced in gaining control over pregnancy and childbirth.

# 6

# Experiences of postnatal care

## Introduction

The unusual amount of attention given to pregnancy and childbirth tends to overshadow the period immediately after birth. In the process, many important aspects of postnatal care and other issues which determine women's adjustment to motherhood are marginalized. Evidence suggests that, once the euphoria of birth is over, the postnatal period can be both emotionally and physically stressful. Many women find it a challenging experience to cope with sleepless nights and the unceasing demands of a baby who needs changing and feeding, as well as the pain of stitches. The nature and level of support in the early weeks after birth can have a major impact on adjustment to motherhood.

In similar vein, a review of the literature on pregnancy and childbirth also reveals a large gap in information about women's experiences of postnatal care. The small number of studies on postnatal care are written largely from the perspective of white women (Oakley 1981; Moss *et al.* 1987; Green *et al.* 1990); there is comparatively little information on South Asian women's experiences. Studies by Dobson (1988) and Woollett and Dosanjh-Matwala (1990b) are, however, exceptions to this general trend.

This chapter examines Gujarati and Bangladeshi women's experiences of postnatal care in hospital and at home within six weeks of birth. It compares and contrasts women's experiences of nursing care, dietary needs, childcare and the nature of support that was available at home. It explores cultural differences in the approach to and expectations of care for mothers and newborn babies.

## Postnatal recovery in hospital

After childbirth it is customary to confine the mother and her baby to the postnatal ward of the maternity hospital for a short period. The length of confinement can vary from just a few hours after delivery to between two and five days depending on the condition of the mother and her baby.

Among the women interviewed, for many first-time mothers but also for some multiparous Bangladeshi women, hospital confinement after childbirth was a new experience. This was particularly the case with Bangladeshi women whose previous childbirth and postnatal experiences were based on home confinement. The following account given by a Bangladeshi maternity liaison worker describes a typical example of events following a home birth in Bangladesh and the six weeks or '40 days' convalescent period:

> As soon as the baby and the afterbirth have been delivered the *dai* (village midwife) or one of the female relatives cuts the cord. The baby is given a bath straight away so that a male member of the family can perform a prayer ceremony called *azan*. The mother meanwhile is carried to the bathroom and given a complete wash by her mother or her mother-in-law. If a mother is weak the bath is delayed for a couple of hours. In the first hours of baby's birth, the baby is given a little water sweetened with honey and the baby is breastfed after the mother has had her bath. For the duration of 40 days after delivery the mother and her baby are isolated because the mother is considered 'unclean' while she is producing discharge.
>
> (Bangladeshi maternity liaison worker)

A similar period of confinement for 40 days or *sawa maheena* is also observed by many Gujarati women. Although the practice of confining the mother to the bed for about ten days and within her house for 40 days may appear restrictive, there are logical explanations to account for such traditions. For example, the 40-day confinement not only gives the mother exemption from the labour of all household chores but the mother is also given additional nutritious foods to aid her recovery. This practice is not unique to Bangladeshi or Gujarati women as similar traditions are noted in other ethnic groups in South Asia. There is evidence to suggest that a similar practice is also observed among parturient mothers in many other countries including China, Latin American and African countries (Pillsbury 1978; MacCormack 1982).

In contrast, few Gujarati women were familiar with home births. However, as will become evident, they shared similar beliefs and practices with regards to dietary restrictions, ceremonial rituals and the 40-day confinement after childbirth. Although many Gujarati women had adopted western attitudes towards childbirth, they were nevertheless expected by mothers-in-law or mothers to observe the ceremonial rituals and dietary customs after childbirth. In following the progress of the women from pregnancy to birth it is apparent that the women's experiences of pregnancy and childbirth were simultaneously subjected to the influences of female relatives and medical professionals, and the only time when female relatives lost their influence was the time the women spent in the labour ward. However, after the birth of a baby, the influence of female relatives was re-established to ensure that the confinement of the mother and baby followed traditional patterns according to family customs.

The care offered to mothers in the hospital thus contrasted sharply with the traditional post-partum care given to women in South Asian communities where the final act of birth does not signal the end of the special status the women have enjoyed during their pregnancies. Instead they continue to receive personal care from their female relatives in the first few weeks after birth.

## Experiences of nursing care in the hospital

Although some Gujarati and Bangladeshi women made positive comments about their postnatal care, on the whole their opinions were ambiguous and in many respects were more closely aligned with the findings of studies of white women (Oakley 1979). For example, many Gujarati and Bangladeshi women reported that they were generally satisfied with the care, but restricted their comments to: 'It was fine' or, 'They took good care of me.' A number of inferences could be drawn from their responses – either that the women's affirmative remarks were, indeed, a true reflection of their views, confirming the findings of Windsor-Richards and Gillies (1988), or that the women were reluctant to give their honest opinion for the fear of appearing ungrateful.

It is important that a certain amount of caution is exercised in the interpretation of women's views of maternity care. For example, although not all women were entirely satisfied with the care they had received, it was evident from their comments that they were unwilling to express their disappointment because they did not wish to appear ungracious:

> I had to write comments to describe how I felt about giving birth in my local hospital. I filled in the questionnaire stating my bad treatment but in the end I tore it up. I couldn't hand in my form . . . I felt bad because I had given birth to my son in this hospital.
>
> (Gujarati mother, second pregnancy)

Ambiguous feelings about postnatal care were also apparent in the reluctance of some Bangladeshi women to offer opinions about their experiences. Some claimed that, since it was their first baby, they did not know what to expect and therefore were not in a position to judge the quality of care they had received. A small number of Bangladeshi women, however, explained that one of the main challenges facing them was to survive in an alien environment where no one spoke their language. Although they accepted that giving birth in hospital would be very different from giving birth at home, they had, nevertheless, expected that the nurse's role and the level of support would be on a par with the role performed by their female relatives:

> My mother-in-law and my aunt helped me a lot when my other children were born in my country. They helped me with everything. I was not allowed to get up . . . they took care of everything. I had this baby at X Hospital last month. After delivery, I felt weak and the baby was crying but no one came to help. After a long time a nurse came and said something but I didn't understand . . . She helped me get out of the bed and took me to the baby and left me. I thought she did not help me because I could not speak her language.
>
> (Bangladeshi mother, fifth pregnancy)

When faced with a different system of managing postnatal care, it was not surprising that some women were puzzled by the attitudes and behaviour of the nurses towards them. For instance, women who expected to have complete bed rest in the first few days after delivery found the hospital practice of getting a mother back on her feet within a few hours of birth unacceptable. Although there are good reasons for encouraging women to become mobile, women who were not aware of this practice found it very difficult to understand why the nurses insisted that they should visit the bathroom within six hours of delivery. For example, discussion with a Bangladeshi maternity liaison worker revealed that sometimes the mothers' reluctance to get out of bed was misunderstood by the nursing staff:

> Many Bangladeshi women feel that the nurses are very unfeeling towards them because they are forced to get up when they are feeling very weak. The nurses think that the Bangladeshi women are lazy and dirty as they are slow to get up and use the bathroom. In Bangladesh a newly delivered mother is not expected to get up immediately; instead her female relatives will carry her to the bathroom and give her a complete wash.
>
> (Bangladeshi maternity liaison worker)

From this and similar accounts reported in other studies (Ahmed and Watt 1986; Woollett and Dosanjh-Matwala 1990b) it is evident that the current management of postnatal care in hospital, which places greater emphasis on the speedy rehabilitation of mothers and the need to establish 'bonding' between mother and baby, diminishes the social significance of childbirth and integration of mother and new baby within the family. MacFarlane's (1984) critical analysis of literature on the concept of 'bonding' argues that the importance attached to the concept is misguided and inappropriate. Not only are there wide variations in the way individual mothers respond to their newborn baby, but the notion of 'bonding' in some cultures would be interpreted as an exclusive relationship and would go against the grain of social and cultural beliefs about family and kinship ties (Dobson 1988).

In Britain, the treatment of pregnancy and childbirth places greater emphasis on the role of medicine and medical experts. This pathological approach to the management of pregnancy and childbirth treats women as if they are all potentially at risk by subjecting them to a series of tests and medical examinations. However, once the baby is delivered there is a marked shift in attitudes and treatment which leaves many mothers feeling bewildered and aggrieved by the apparent lack of interest in their welfare. Although there are good reasons for encouraging women to make a speedy recovery and take responsibility for the care of their babies, the sudden change in attitude often does not take into account the fact that individual women take different lengths of time to overcome the after-effects of drugs used in labour or to recover from any surgical procedures they may have undergone. A number of Gujarati women who had difficult labours and deliveries were upset by the offhand manner by which their concerns were met by the staff. For example, one of the commonest complaints made by some Gujarati women was that they could not understand why they were paid less attention once the delivery was over:

> I was attended to by two doctors, a midwife and a paediatrician before my son was born but once the delivery was over I had to wait a long time before my cut was stitched up . . . After I was stitched up I was left unattended for four hours in the labour ward. No one seemed to be bothered about me. I was finally taken to the postnatal ward. By this time I was really starving, as I had not eaten for two days. I asked for some sandwiches but they never materialized. I was feeling very weak and faint from lack of food and I felt very neglected as if no one cared for me.
>
> (Gujarati mother, first pregnancy)

Another Gujarati mother claimed that the nurses' attitudes towards women were based on stereotypes about women who were already mothers and consequently multiparous women received less attention regardless of the fact that their previous experience of childbirth did not give them immunity against complicated labours or make it easier to cope with subsequent births:

> I was left unattended for some time after I was transferred from the labour ward. I was in a lot of pain because the forceps were not applied properly. The first time I called for an assistant to go to the bathroom the nurse told me off for ringing the bell and for making a fuss about my stitches. She promised to bring some ice to reduce the swelling and again I had to wait a long time for it. When a nurse finally brought the ice for me she didn't explain how I should use it. As I had never used ice before I just sat there wondering what to do because I was afraid of wetting the bed. I was told not to ring the bell for assistance because they were short of staff. I stayed in the hospital for five days thinking I would get more help than I could at home. The attitude of the staff was that second-time mums have previous experience so they just expect you to get on with it but I was in so much pain I needed more help.
>
> (Gujarati mother, second pregnancy)

Many women found it difficult to adjust to the fact that, although the attention they received in the antenatal period implied that their care during pregnancy was a medical emergency, within hours of delivery they became a 'nuisance' to the nursing staff. Women who had surgical interventions, like episiotomies or Caesarean sections, felt that the nursing staff did not appreciate how much pain they were experiencing. Some felt that they were made to feel guilty for occupying a hospital bed when all they had done was give birth and were certainly not 'sick'. Although a shortage of staff was a contributory factor, some women felt that the zeal with which some nurses set about getting them back on their feet did not give due consideration to their vulnerability in the postpartum period. A Gujarati mother who had undergone emergency Caesarean section was very upset with the unsympathetic attitude of the nursing staff:

> I did not enjoy my stay in the hospital. At the moment I feel I will never go back to that hospital again. I found it was difficult to manage with my stitches and yet I was expected to get on and do everything myself. Some of the nurses were very rude as well. Because I had a Caesarean section I was finding it difficult to walk back and forth to the special care unit to see my daughter. My stitches were so painful I found it difficult to wheel the breast pump to my room and yet no one helped me. In the morning, if I was resting, the nurses would make rude comments like, 'Are you still sleeping?' as if I was too lazy to get out of bed. I was originally booked in for just two days but as I had a Caesarean section I was not discharged for eleven days.
>
> (Gujarati mother, first pregnancy)

It would seem that women whose perception of postnatal care was determined by their cultural values were confronted with concepts of care which in many respects were unlike anything they had experienced before. Asian women in Woollett and Dosanjh-Matwala's (1990b) and Dobson's (1988) studies raised similar concerns about the mismatch in expectations and disappointment about postnatal care. While the women used different strategies to mediate between two parallel systems of care during their pregnancy, their options for manoeuvring between two systems were drastically reduced after admission into hospital for labour and delivery. The differences in expectations became most evident in the women's struggle to comprehend the totally different approach to managing the care of parturient mothers. Communication and language barriers seriously undermined the quality of care. The negative attitudes and behaviour of nursing staff also affected the women's experience of their hospital stay. Minority ethnic women of childbearing age have the most need of health care services for themselves and for their children and yet racism remains a major barrier in the National Health Service. While accounts of racist attitudes and behaviour encountered by minority ethnic women may go unnoticed or, worse, not be taken seriously, Bowler's (1993) investigation of midwifery and obstetric practices leaves little doubt about the existence of overt and covert racism practised by midwives and obstetric staff.

## Dietary requirements after childbirth

Although there is a huge variation in dietary habits and preferences, the importance of a well-balanced diet in pregnancy and after childbirth is recognized across all cultures. In addition, it is widely acknowledged that good nutrition in the first few weeks after childbirth is very important for a mother to regain her strength and to establish successful breastfeeding (NCT 1992; Worthington-Roberts and Williams 1993). The issue of the psycho-social and therapeutic significance of dietary beliefs and practices in the management of pregnancy, discussed in Chapter 4, resurfaced as an important theme in the postnatal interviews. Much of the discussion centred around their concern about the inadequacy and inappropriateness of meals provided in the hospital and the importance of their traditional diet after childbirth.

The current practice of managing rehabilitation of parturient mothers has reduced the length of time during which women are confined to maternity hospital. However, some women are confined for a longer period in hospital if there are complications in pregnancy or if they have had a difficult labour and delivery. On average, the Bangladeshi and Gujarati women spent three to five days in hospital, but in some cases their stay had been extended to two or more weeks when making a slow recovery after surgical interventions. It was, therefore, not surprising that access to adequate and appropriate meals had a considerable impact on their experience of postnatal care in hospital.

Many hospitals in Britain have realized the importance of providing hospital meals to meet the cultural and religious needs of patients. However, for a variety of reasons, the provision of hospital meals remains a cause of concern to many patients. The hospital where a majority of the Gujarati women gave birth was operating a policy which did not allow women to receive any meals prepared at home. At the second hospital where a majority of Bangladeshi women gave birth, the women were encouraged to receive food from home because the range of food in the hospital was inadequate to meet the dietary requirements of Muslim women. A number of these women were also upset by the lack of sensitivity in understanding their needs as some vegetarian meals on the menu were labelled as 'halal'. The term 'halal' (meaning 'permitted') is normally used only in connection with meat which has been obtained from an animal slaughtered in accordance with the Islamic faith. Consequently, only vegetarian options were available to those who wished for halal food. This hospital actively encouraged women to receive food from home, if they found hospital food unpalatable or unacceptable on religious grounds, providing an ideal solution and absolving them of their responsibility. In the process, however, responsibility was transferred to the women's families. As we shall see, for many Bangladeshi women and their hard-pressed families, taking food into hospital was fraught with difficulties.

The women's views about the hospital food were divided. A small number of women, mostly Gujarati women, who were non-vegetarian said that they enjoyed the hospital food because they were able to choose vegetarian and non-vegetarian meals and therefore had more varied meals:

> I must say I enjoyed the hospital food because I was always hungry. It was also nice to be able to eat food which I had not cooked myself and besides I was able to choose different food; sometimes I had English food and sometimes I had vegetarian food.
>
> (Gujarati mother, second pregnancy)

On the other hand, for a variety of reasons, an overwhelmingly large number of the Gujarati and Bangladeshi mothers claimed that they were disappointed with the food they had been offered in hospital. Many Gujarati women felt that, although vegetarian meals were provided, not enough effort was made to ensure they were appropriate and adequate to meet the needs of mothers who were trying to establish breastfeeding:

> I thought the hospital food was terrible! . . . the portions were very small, not enough for a breastfeeding mother. I did not feel satisfied with what I had. They also did not present the meals with any imagination; sometimes we were served the same bean curry for lunch and supper. I was not keen to eat too many beans because it causes indigestion.
>
> (Gujarati mother, second pregnancy)

Other women complained that the system of offering a menu a day in advance did not work in practice. In some cases, the women did not get the meals they had selected and had to experience considerable delay before they were given something to eat:

> As I am a vegetarian it made it difficult to get decent meals. I only had three meals and each time the staff had to search for a vegetarian meal and often I was kept waiting before they could find something for me. By the time the food was brought to me it was cold. It was very irritating but I had no choice as I was starving. My husband was very angry and wanted to complain but I felt it was not worth it.
>
> (Gujarati mother, second pregnancy)

While the Gujarati women were able to offer their opinions about the quality and quantity of food, many Bangladeshi women felt that they were not in a position to express their views on hospital food because they had been unwilling to accept meals which did not satisfy their religious requirements. The only food the women were able to comment upon was bread and tea: 'The nurse used to give me bread and milk but I do not like the milk in this country . . . it tasted not very nice. I used to drink tea' (Bangladeshi mother, third pregnancy).

The unavailability of food which met Muslim women's religious requirements was a real cause of concern for many Bangladeshi women who were detained in the hospital for more than a week. Many felt that they were left with a stark choice – either rely on their husbands to bring food from home or manage on bread and tea since the only other items on the menu offered as a vegetarian choice were cheese or eggs. Indeed, many Bangladeshi women chose to survive on bread and tea until their husbands brought food from home:

> The only thing I could eat was bread and tea. My husband brought rice and fish curry from home when he visited me in the evening. He couldn't manage any other times . . . how could he? He also had to look after my other children.
>
> (Bangladeshi mother, fifth pregnancy)

For some Bangladeshi women, the vegetarian meals offered on the menu were also unacceptable because they were concerned about the method of food preparation and handling and believed that in the hospital kitchen cross-contamination of food was unavoidable:

> I am a devout Muslim and because my religion does not allow me to eat certain things, I am not happy to eat hospital food. I am not sure how it is possible for a hospital to prepare meals for so many patients and keep food separate for Muslim patients. I was not happy to eat hospital food . . . I had to wait for my husband. He used to bring food from home when he visited me in the evening.
>
> (Bangladeshi mother, first pregnancy)

However, since many Bangladeshi women were relatively new to this country and did not have an extensive network of friends and relatives to care for them, this often meant a long wait for food to be brought to them. Many husbands could not take time off work in the middle of the day or had responsibilities for other children at home.

In many respects the Gujarati women appeared in an enviable position. Not only did their local hospital make some effort to provide a choice of Indian vegetarian meals on the menu each day, but they also had an extensive social network of female relatives at hand to provide both practical and emotional support while they were in hospital. However, as is evident, not all women were content with the hospital vegetarian food and the ban on mothers receiving food prepared at home became a source of deep unhappiness. While some managed to avoid being detected eating food brought from home, those who were either found eating home-cooked food or whose relatives requested permission to bring food were reminded about the hospital policy: 'My sister-in-law wanted to bring some food for me because I was feeling very weak after the delivery. When she went to get permission from the ward sister she was told that patients were not allowed to eat any food brought from home' (Gujarati mother, third pregnancy).

To discourage relatives from bringing food from home some mothers were told that home-cooked food was banned because it brings infection into the hospital. Gujarati women who were offered this explanation were deeply offended, as this comment suggests:

> I found the hospital food unappetizing. My husband brought some food from home, which my sister-in-law had cooked. When the nurse saw me eating the food he had brought she told him off. She told my husband that I would suffer from stomach pain because I was eating food brought from home. She made me feel that our food was bad. What made it worse for me was that I was confined in the hospital for nearly two weeks.
>
> (Gujarati mother, first pregnancy)

For many Gujarati women and their families, the ban was an unjustified imposition and showed a lack of respect and understanding of values and beliefs about childbirth which were different from their own. While pregnancy is considered to be a 'hot' state (see earlier discussion in Chapter 4, page 50), the period of '40 days' or six weeks after childbirth constitutes a 'cold' state. During each phase, the fine balance of bodily humours is maintained by dietary control, i.e. during pregnancy 'cold' foods are recommended and after childbirth 'hot' foods are recommended. For example, the traditional diet after childbirth consisted of foods containing 'hot' properties such as milk products, wholegrain cereals and leafy vegetables, including a sweetmeat, variously referred to as *katlu*, *Penjerri* or *kalo jeera barta*, which is prepared for mothers after parturition (Homans 1983; Woollett and Dosanjh-Matwala 1990b; Spiro 1994). This sweetmeat consists of wholemeal wheat flour, nuts, many different spices and unrefined sugar. It is believed to be highly nutritious and has special properties to aid recovery and establish lactation. Some of the spices, such as dried root ginger in the sweetmeat, are believed to have special properties to help strengthen the pelvic joints and speed up the involution of the womb while nuts provide much needed protein for the mother and her baby. The high content of fibres in the diet also helps to prevent constipation. In addition, a drink made with an infusion of herbs such as dill seeds is given to the mother to cleanse her system and to increase milk supply (Raja 1993; Schott and Henley 1996).

Apart from the inherent nutritional and healing qualities of the traditional diet, the preparation and consumption of the sweetmeat is vested with symbolic significance. For example, for mothers and mothers-in-law the preparation of the sweetmeat constituted an act of public recognition of the new status of their daughter or daughter-in-law and facilitated the integration of new mother and baby into the folds of the family. The giving and receiving of the sweetmeat was also an act of strengthening and renewing social bonds between family members. As will become clear later, the failure of a family to discharge their obligations to a new mother was interpreted by some women and by the wider community as a sign of neglect or an affront to the mother. As the discussion in the next chapter suggests, older women who see themselves as the guardians of cultural traditions feel duty bound to ensure that their daughters and daughters-in-law follow the dietary advice:

> I didn't like the hospital food at all. I didn't enjoy the vegetarian or the non-vegetarian meals. I couldn't receive food from home. My mother-in-law was annoyed because she could not bring the traditional food which she felt I should be eating after childbirth. The other Indian ladies in my ward used to receive food from home and eat it secretly behind the drawn curtains. I wasn't prepared to do that. The only thing I was able to have was *rab* [thick liquid food made from wholemeal flour, spices and unrefined brown sugar].
>
> (Gujarati mother, first pregnancy)

Although some relatives reluctantly accepted the ban on home cooked food, other women and their relatives were prepared to defy the hospital rules because they had a strong belief in the beneficial effects of traditional foods. One such mother explained how she got round the hospital rule:

> The food in the hospital has not improved at all since I had my first baby three years ago. They tend to give you a lot of potatoes, which I believe are not good for you in the early days after delivery. The rice and curry were all mixed up and it didn't look very appetizing. I used to receive food from home although it was strictly forbidden. My mother-in-law used to bring food at visiting time and while I was surrounded by my family I used to eat the food then because the nurses did not come to check during visiting hour.
>
> (Gujarati mother, second pregnancy)

The strength of beliefs in the value of the traditional diet was evident from the fact that many Gujarati women claimed that they were offered traditional foods after they were discharged from the hospital. A Gujarati explained:

> I have been having traditional food since the birth of my baby. My mother-in-law used to smuggle food into hospital. After I came home my mother-in-law cooked separate food for me for four more weeks. My mother also brought some *katlu* for me. I feel it is important to eat our traditional foods because it helps with recovery. I am now eating the same food as the rest of the family but I still avoid heavy pulses such as beans, which would give colic to my baby.
>
> (Gujarati mother, first pregnancy)

After the Bangladeshi women were discharged from the hospital they did not mention any special diet except the avoidance of meat, especially beef, which they considered to be 'hot' and not recommended after childbirth: 'For a couple of weeks after I came home I did not eat any meat or any spicy food but instead I ate more fish and vegetables' (Bangladeshi mother, seventh pregnancy). Although a special diet was also believed to be necessary after childbirth, very few Bangladeshi women had mothers or mothers-in-law living in this country who could prepare special food for them.

It is thus evident that, for the Gujarati and Bangladeshi women, cultural and religious beliefs about diet and the need to observe the dietary beliefs based on the concept of 'hot' and 'cold' foods was an important part of postnatal recovery as was also the case during pregnancy. However, this ability to engage in culturally appropriate practices was dependent on numerous variables, including the presence of other family members to facilitate cultural compliance.

For many women hospitalization for childbirth involved having to accept hospital meals which clashed with their religious and cultural beliefs. Although the local hospitals had made some attempt to cater for the dietary needs of Asian women, they had clearly failed to meet their requirements. The rigid application of a hospital food policy, without prior consultation with the community concerned, was interpreted by many women as demeaning and disrespectful to cultural beliefs. On the other hand, a hospital which appeared to have more liberal attitudes towards patients receiving food from home had failed to meet its obligations to provide culturally appropriate meals for a large number of Muslim patients.

For Asian, and in particular Gujarati, women, the traditional diet after childbirth seemed to play a dual purpose. It was used both as a part of the healing mechanism after childbirth and, for the relatives, as a ritual which they were expected to fulfil to show their respect and affection for a member of their family who had just given birth. The fact that many Gujarati women expressed a strong desire to receive food recommended by their relatives seems to suggest an interesting transformation in their attitudes towards traditional diet and dietary restrictions in pregnancy. It was evident that the same women who had found it irksome to observe their female relatives' dietary advice in pregnancy were upset when they were prevented from receiving food prepared by their relatives. Indeed, in a small number of cases, relatives' failure to discharge their obligations was interpreted by the women as a sign of disrespect. The remarkable reversal in their attitudes towards traditional diet is difficult to explain and one can only speculate that their desire to receive food specially prepared by their relatives was an acknowledgement of mutual obligation: the birth of a baby became a source of celebration rather than conflict. Another explanation could be that the women did not have to deal with the conflicting advice about diet which they had faced in pregnancy as the professional interest in the nutritional status of women was no longer a major concern for them. The fact that the women's relatives were interested in their welfare may have heightened the importance of traditional diet. Additionally, the obvious dissatisfaction with hospital food may have removed any doubt women may have had about the benefits of traditional diet.

## Care of the baby – choice of feeding methods

For a period after the Second World War breastfeeding became less popular but, since the health professionals and mothers have come to recognize the benefits offered by breastmilk, breastfeeding is enjoying a renaissance. This is apparent from the steady growth in breastfeeding rates in the UK in the last ten years (Foster *et al.* 1997). However, Foster *et al.* point out that this growth in the incidence of breastfeeding is unevenly spread across different ethnic groups and is governed by the socio-economic, education, age and ethnic background of mothers. Mothers who had been in full-time education up to the age of 14, mothers who were over the age of 18 and those belonging to a higher socio-economic group were more likely to breastfeed their baby for the first four or five months. A separate and parallel survey of infant feeding practices in South Asian families living in England revealed that although the incidence of breastfeeding among Indian, Pakistani and Bangladeshi mothers was higher than among white mothers, Bangladeshi and Pakistani mothers were more likely than Indian and white mothers to stop breastfeeding altogether within eight weeks of birth (Thomas and Avery 1997). Thomas and Avery (1997) and Ahmet (1990), among others, suggest that the increase in bottle-feeding set up an adverse trend for weaning the baby off bottled milk. Given the generally low socio-economic position of many Bangladeshi and Pakistani families in Britain (Modood *et al.* 1997), it is perhaps not very surprising to find that women within these communities give up breastfeeding in the first few weeks of birth.

Traditionally, most women on the Indian subcontinent breastfeed their babies. However, the present generation of childbearing women have grown up in an age when bottle-feeding is actively promoted as a credible alternative to breastmilk in the west and, particularly, in underdeveloped countries. Before powdered baby milk became available pregnant women did not have to consider how they should feed their baby and, in many underdeveloped countries where women cannot afford to buy formula milk, this is still the case. Ahmet (1990), for instance, suggests that for most mothers in Bangladesh, with the exception of affluent mothers, the question of how they should feed their babies does not arise as it is assumed that women have no alternative but to breastfeed their babies. In Britain, pregnant women use a number of external sources of information about infant feeding before making their decision. These sources are antenatal classes, printed literature and female friends and relatives and also knowledge based on previous experience of feeding other children.

When the women were asked about their choice of feeding methods in the prenatal period, almost half the women from both groups had intended to breastfeed only, while most of the others reported that they would supplement breast milk with powdered baby milk. Contrary to expectations, more Gujarati than Bangladeshi women had intended to breastfeed their babies, while Bangladeshi women had stated a stronger preference for combining breastfeeding with bottle-feeding. Thomas and Avery (1997) report similar findings. It is interesting to note that, of the Gujarati women, only two actually decided to bottle-feed. The apparent change in attitudes towards breastfeeding reported by many Bangladeshi women was surprising given that many women had recently arrived from Bangladesh where breastfeeding is the only viable option for most women. This trend is particularly worrying considering that there is evidence to suggest that women who were themselves breastfed were more likely to breastfeed their own babies, as were women who had breastfed a previous child (Thomas and Avery 1997). The explanations for the Bangladeshi women's preference for bottle-feeding were complex and multifaceted. Some of the commonest reasons cited were fear of producing insufficient milk coupled with the idea that, unless bottle-feeding was introduced early, the baby would not get used to it:

> In my country, I did not give tinned milk to my other children. When I came to this country my sister-in-law and my neighbour told me that it is important to get the baby used to the bottle early because when the breastmilk is not enough the baby will accept milk from the bottle without difficulty.
>
> (Bangladeshi mother, fifth pregnancy)

Apart from the anxiety concerning insufficient breastmilk, some women also experienced peer group pressure to introduce supplementary powdered milk. The change in attitude towards breastfeeding was also apparent among Bangladeshi women who had solely breastfed other children in Bangladesh. Six out of eight multipara women who had solely breastfed their other babies for three to four months had planned to use powdered baby milk this time:

> My neighbour had all her children in this country and she told me that bottle-feeding is easier than breastfeeding because you can easily tell how much milk a baby has taken. I am going to give breastmilk and powdered milk . . . that way my baby has both.
>
> (Bangladeshi mother, first pregnancy)

In contrast, many Gujarati women's strong preference for breastfeeding reflected the revival of breastfeeding in the west. Their favourable attitudes were influenced by information they had obtained from parentcraft classes and from printed literature, television and radio programmes: 'I am hoping that I can. After I heard the parentcraft teacher talk about the advantages of breastmilk . . . I would have a go. I found out as much as I can from reading magazines and books before I decided in favour of breastfeeding' (Gujarati mother, first pregnancy).

The positive image of breastfeeding among the Gujarati women was further reflected in the commitment of almost all multiparous women who had intended to breastfeed their second or third baby. The only exceptions were a small number of multiparous Gujarati women who had planned to bottle-feed. It would seem that women who had ambiguous feelings about their pregnancies were more likely to declare a preference for bottle-feeding:

> I breastfed my last two babies. This time I am going to bottle-feed. I just can't see myself breastfeeding this time somehow. I don't

> know . . . everything seems wrong somehow. We hadn't planned it . . . I had even thought of terminating it in the beginning. Now I am worried about all the medicine I had taken [crying] . . . to get rid of the baby. I feel just numb about everything.
>
> (Gujarati mother, third pregnancy)

The generally more favourable attitudes towards bottle-feeding seem to suggest a worrying trend among Bangladeshi women. Other writers (Ahmet 1990; Thomas and Avery 1997) have raised similar concerns about the decline in breastfeeding within the Bangladeshi community. It is particularly unfortunate that an ideal opportunity provided by the example of a positive infant feeding practice, well rooted in the cultural traditions of Bangladesh, is not actively reinforced.

In the follow-up interviews, which took place between four and six weeks after birth, the women were asked about the method of feeding their baby and whether or not this was the choice made before the birth. When the women's responses were compared against the responses they had given during pregnancy, a pattern of infant feeding emerged which contrasted sharply with their original intentions. For example, four weeks after birth, only a small number of women, predominately Gujarati, were solely breastfeeding. All but one of the Bangladeshi women who had intended to breastfeed only were combining breastfeeding with bottle-feeding within six weeks of the birth. The most marked change in feeding practice was thus observed among the Bangladeshi women, a majority of whom had become accustomed to supplementing breastfeeding with artificial baby milk. Although a similar decline in breastfeeding was also evident among the Gujarati women, the drop was less marked. A small number of Gujarati women who had intended to bottle-feed had not changed their minds after the birth, with the exception of one multiparous Gujarati woman who wanted to terminate her pregnancy:

> When he was born I didn't feel anything, just relieved that it was all over. He was born under the effects of pethidine so he just slept and didn't even cry. I was a bit worried. I had decided to use the bottle . . . but then I changed my mind and decided to feed him myself . . . well . . . I felt so bad.
>
> (Gujarati mother, third pregnancy)

On closer examination, it would seem that the increase in bottle feeding followed a set pattern. For example, women who had planned solely to breastfeed continued breastfeeding, but only partially, whereas those who had intended to supplement breastfeeding with artificial milk had given up breastfeeding altogether. In many respects, the infant feeding practice reflected the trends reported for white women (Thomson 1989).

Nevertheless, the sharp increase in the number of women who were only partially breastfeeding and those who had stopped breastfeeding altogether is a matter of concern, given that so few women had expressed doubt about their ability to breastfeed or had envisaged potential problems in the antenatal interview. It is widely accepted that the management of labour and delivery and postnatal care can have serious implications for the establishment of successful breastfeeding (Messenger-Davies 1986). For example, factors such as the inflexible hospital routine, the lack of appropriate support and encouragement from nursing staff, slow recovery of the mother after delivery, especially if surgical interventions and drugs were used in labour, and the separation of mother and baby after birth can all effectively undermine any attempt to establish successful breastfeeding:

> I had planned to breastfeed my baby but it all went wrong from the beginning. I had a Caesarean section and my baby was admitted to the baby unit. I did not get any help. I was told to express my milk with a mechanical breast pump, which I had to bring from another room. Because of my painful stitches I found it difficult to manoeuvre the pump but no one was prepared to help. The other problem was that I was given so much conflicting advice about feeding from different members of the staff that I used to get quite confused.
>
> (Gujarati mother, first pregnancy)

In another case, a Bangladeshi mother explained that she was unable to continue with breastfeeding due to lack of support. Thomas and Avery (1997) report that, of the South Asian mothers, Bangladeshi mothers were least likely to receive help and advice with their feeding problems. Some women claimed that they had never stayed in a hospital before and found the atmosphere in the hospital very unfriendly. They were unable to ask for help because the nurses could not speak their language:

> I wanted to breastfeed in the beginning but I could not manage it . . . if my mother or my sister were with me they would have helped. I found it difficult to feed the baby but I could not ask for help because I felt embarrassed to ask anyone. I then decided to bottle-feed.
>
> (Bangladeshi mother, first pregnancy)

Evidence from literature on childbirth suggests that the lack of reassurance and encouragement in the early weeks after birth often discouraged women from persevering with initial difficulties with breastfeeding. In many respects, the difficulties recounted by the two groups with breastfeeding were similar to those reported by many other British women (Eiser and Eiser 1985; Bhopal and White 1993). However, language barriers, different dietary requirements, unfamiliarity with hospital routines and the unsympathetic attitudes of nurses created additional difficulties for the women: 'Because of my stitches I could not sit on a chair to feed my baby. I was told off for feeding my son in the bed. I often had to feed him standing up. I thought they [nurses] would understand . . . but no, they did not seem to care' (Gujarati mother, second pregnancy).

The customary taboo against feeding colostrum (Ahmet 1990) to a newborn baby also resulted in lack of support for women who wanted to delay breastfeeding immediately after birth. Colostrum, together with other bodily discharges, is believed by some Asian women to be a source of pollution and is therefore considered harmful to newborn babies. Unfortunately, the belief about colostrum is often misconstrued by nursing staff as an indication of Asian women's lack of interest in breastfeeding. According to Bangladeshi maternity liaison workers, women ready to start breastfeeding were given little encouragement:

> Many Bangladeshi women, like other women, face similar problems with breastfeeding in the first few days. Just because a few women are reluctant to feed baby colostrum, the hospital staff assume that it's a common practice and even those women who do not have any strong feeling about colostrum are denied support. Some older women in the community consider colostrum to be actually bad for the baby, some women believe that it is not good enough for the baby because it looks watery.
>
> (Bangladeshi maternity liaison worker)

The women's experience of infant feeding suggests that there are implications for improving access to information in the antenatal and postnatal period. Since infant feeding practices adopted in the early weeks of a baby's life could later undermine attempts to wean a child on to traditional diets, it is essential that women get all the support they need after childbirth. To ensure that the information on infant feeding reaches all women, the health education message should take into account the linguistic and cultural diversity of the Asian communities. In addition, since many women expressed anxiety about insufficient breastmilk, emphasis should be placed on the need for a balanced diet during and after childbirth and suggestions for ways to increase the supply of breastmilk should be made available through appropriate channels.

## Postnatal confinement at home: family support and ceremonial rituals

Traditionally an Asian mother who has just delivered a baby relies on her relations to provide care for herself and her baby. Since childbirth and the few weeks immediately afterwards are believed by many Asian people to be an 'unclean' state, the mother is restricted to the confines of her house for a period of 40 days or six weeks. During this period she is also excused from household work and especially anything to do with food preparation while she is 'unclean'. This practice is shared by many other cultures round the world (MacCormack 1982; Blanchet 1984). Although it is restrictive, it ensures that the mother gets all the rest she needs since she is not allowed to enter the cooking area or participate in household chores. In Britain, hospitalization of childbirth means that the isolation ritual only applies after the mother is discharged from the hospital.

It is also a practice among Asian mothers to return to their parental homes in the last weeks of pregnancy, where they stay for the birth and for at least six weeks immediately after the birth. Although this custom is observed largely for the first pregnancy only, it is not unheard of for multipara mothers to return to their parents' home for rest after the baby is a few weeks old.

Because of practical difficulties of keeping this tradition alive, a token visit is made to the parental home by Asian mothers, albeit in a modified form: some women go back for a few days or weeks to their parental home after the six-week 'unclean' period is over. Nevertheless, for many women migration to Britain has resulted in the fragmentation of kinship networks and the loss of the traditional sources of support during and after childbirth. In addition, the hospitalization of birth has meant that women are expected to give birth in the local hospital and have to rely solely on their husband's family for support after childbirth instead of their own parents or relations.

Although it was traditional for women to return to their parental home for childbirth, the women interviewed reported that the visit could only take place provided permission was granted by their husbands and, in some cases, the arrangement had to be negotiated with their in-laws. The delicate nature of the negotiation was evident from the difficulties some women encountered:

> Although my mother-in-law had agreed that I could go to my parents' house for *sawa mahino* [period equivalent to a month and a quarter], she [mother-in-law] only allowed me to stay for just two weeks. My mother and I were really upset but we couldn't do anything about it.
> (Gujarati mother, first pregnancy)

However, some women experienced little difficulty. This arrangement was easier to negotiate if the women's parents lived locally, in which case the women were able to go directly to their parents' home after they were discharged:

> When I was discharged from the hospital, I went back home with my parents, as it is our tradition. It gave me time to get to know my baby because I didn't have any housework to do. I also got a lot of rest. My mother used to do everything for me. All I did was to feed the baby.
> (Gujarati mother, first pregnancy)

On the whole, the Gujarati women were more likely than Bangladeshi women to have relatives nearby and to receive support from their relatives, however this was not always the case. These women had little choice about observing the taboo related to parturient women and had to disregard the beliefs about the 40-day rest period:

> I only stayed in hospital for two days because I have no one to look after my other two children. I have been doing everything myself since

> I returned from the hospital. Fortunately my invalid mother-in-law is not staying with me at the moment so I can just about cope but when she returns it will be difficult to manage as I will have to look after her as well.
>
> (Gujarati mother, third pregnancy)

It was evident that the lack of support affected both groups of women to varying degrees. However, Bangladeshi women appeared to be most affected by the lack of support from their own natal family and had to manage without any support: 'In this country it is very difficult to manage without help. In my country I used to go to my mother's house and she used to help me a lot. I have nobody to help me in this country. My husband doesn't help me because he thinks I should be able to manage' (Bangladeshi mother, sixth pregnancy).

The women who appeared to have the least amount of help at home were the women who were living in the nuclear family. Bangladeshi women who did not have any relatives in this country had to rely mostly on their husbands or older children: 'As my eldest daughter is fourteen years old she helps me a lot now. She looks after the baby – she feeds and changes the baby for me. My husband also helps me with my other children so I manage somehow' (Bangladeshi mother, sixth pregnancy).

According to a Bangladeshi maternity liaison worker, the lack of support is often overlooked by health professionals who assume that all Asian women live in a joint family and therefore do not require help from other sources:

> Some of the older family members are still living in Bangladesh so many families are nuclear. A vast majority of the women who have settled here have no immediate family support other than distant relatives. The health professionals are misguided in assuming that in case of trouble we can rely on the extended family support and they don't have to do anything for us.
>
> (Bangladeshi maternity liaison worker)

Once the initial excitement of childbirth is over, most women need time to recover their strength and adjust to the demands of a new baby. The quality and quantity of practical and emotional support available to women at this time is clearly important for women in making a successful transition to motherhood (Oakley 1992; Woollett *et al.* 1995; Kearns *et al.* 1997). However, the women's access to support depended on how comfortable they felt about accepting help from relatives. One of the most frequently mentioned sources of support was from the women's own natal family. This was also the case with many women whose parents were in Bangladesh, indicating that there was not only a greater expectation of support from this source but also fewer problems with acceptance of this support:

> I felt more comfortable with my mum. It also gave her a chance to look after me and be with my baby. I could only stay with her for two weeks. It is so different being with your own mother. I don't have to

> lift a finger. She made sure I had everything and even helped to look after the baby so that I could rest. I would have preferred to stay a few more weeks at my mother's house.
>
> (Gujarati mother, first pregnancy)

A difference in the expectation and acceptance of support was evident from the women who had to rely on their husbands' families. The women who received help from their husbands' families claimed that they did not get the rest they would have liked as they felt obliged to help with housework:

> I have found it very difficult to cope. I am feeling very emotional and sometimes I feel very depressed. It is hard to look after a new baby – she takes up all my time. I am expected to do all the housework because my mother-in-law believes that it is good to be active and get back to normal as soon as possible. My mother-in-law cooked for me for a week and now she leaves it all to me.
>
> (Gujarati mother, first pregnancy)

Compared with the constraints which many women experienced as a result of the restrictions during pregnancy (see Chapter 4, pages 57–8), restrictions after childbirth appeared to be less objectionable. However, the restriction which required women to remain confined to the home for 40 days was unacceptable to some women. A majority of Bangladeshi women did not find this a problem because they did not have their in-laws to impose such restrictions. However, those who were accustomed to the purdah restriction were happy for their husbands to go shopping and deal with any other business. Some Gujarati women, on the other hand, felt that this restriction did not serve any useful purpose other than to give some members of their husband's family control over them. A Gujarati mother who was prevented from visiting her parents remarked:

> I am not allowed to go anywhere except the clinic for six weeks. I feel as if I am in a jail. I would like to go and stay with my brother but my husband's sister does not approve because he lives in East London. Although she [sister-in-law] does not live with us she has a lot of power and lays down rules for us. I went out yesterday to do some shopping but told my sister-in-law that I had an appointment at the clinic. I do not like to deceive anyone but I don't see why I shouldn't go out.
>
> (Gujarati mother, first pregnancy)

## Summary

One of the major issues to emerge from the accounts of the women's postpartum care is that both Gujarati and Bangladeshi women were dissatisfied with the care they had received during their brief stay in hospital.

A majority of the women had spent at least three days or more in hospital. Their dissatisfaction therefore has implications for a greater understanding of the needs and expectations of the women who come from different cultures.

The main cause of dissatisfaction was partly due to the change in attitude of the nursing staff towards the women after they were admitted into the postnatal ward and partly because many women's perceptions of postnatal care were based on the traditional approach. Many Bangladeshi and Gujarati women were at a loss to understand why they merited less attention from the medical staff as soon as delivery was over when during their pregnancy they were treated as if they were ill. It was particularly confusing for Bangladeshi women who expected the same kind of care and attention they were accustomed to receiving from their female relatives.

The lack of appropriate meals in hospital was another issue which affected the women's perception of the care they had received. It would seem that, despite good intentions on the part of one hospital to cater for particular dietary requirements, rigid restrictions prohibiting women from receiving food from home were counterproductive. Many Gujarati women found that the hospital meals were inadequate and did not take into account the significance of traditional foods for the women or their relatives. Although Bangladeshi women did not have similar restrictions on receiving food from home, hospital meals failed to meet religious dietary requirements, with serious implications for nursing mothers, especially as some women may spend two or more weeks in hospital.

It was worrying that the number of women who had intended to breastfeed their babies fell after birth. It was particularly significant in the case of the Bangladeshi women who had begun to doubt their ability to produce sufficient milk for their babies. The fact that Bangladeshi women had not abandoned breastfeeding altogether suggests that positive reinforcement and support in the first weeks of birth would give women confidence in their ability to supply the needs of their babies without resorting to artificial baby milk. Gujarati women, on the other hand, were influenced by the current popularity enjoyed by breastfeeding. This was reflected in the number who had planned to breastfeed and who were only giving breastmilk after birth. However, the fact that some Gujarati women had also introduced powdered milk indicates that support in the first few weeks after birth is crucial.

Finally, emotional and practical support provided by the family is very important for the women to make a full recovery after childbirth. In the case of Gujarati women, the majority were fortunate in having their female relatives to provide support after they were discharged from the hospital. However, it would be wrong to assume that Asian women do not require support from the health carers because they live in joint households. The experiences of Bangladeshi women indicated that many suffer from isolation and lack traditional support because their families have been fragmented after their migration to Britain.

## Annotated bibliography

Pillsbury, B.L.K. (1978) Doing the month: confinement and convalescence of Chinese women after childbirth, *Social Science and Medicine*, 12: 11–22.

While this is not a recent paper, the author explores ideas and beliefs about postnatal care and the importance of observing a set of rules about proscriptions and prescriptions after childbirth. She describes the psychological and practical relevance of postnatal confinement in Chinese culture.

Thomas, M. and Avery, V. (1997) *Infant Feeding in Asian Families: A Survey Carried Out in England by the Social Survey Division of ONS on Behalf of the Department of Health*. London: The Stationery Office.

This survey provides an account of infant feeding practices in Asian families in England and Wales, highlighting the enormous differences in infant feeding practices between Indian, Pakistani and Bangladeshi mothers. The survey reports on the incidence and prevalence of breastfeeding, on access to information and advice and on the reasons why mothers give up breastfeeding.

Woollett, A. and Dosanjh-Matwala, N. (1990b) Postnatal care: the attitudes and experiences of Asian women in east London, *Midwifery*, 6: 178–84.

This paper compares the experiences of postnatal care of Asian and white women. The discussion focuses on differences in ideologies around the care of mothers and babies, the nature of early mother–infant relations and the difficulties it creates for Asian women.

# 7

# Negotiating pregnancy and childbirth within extended households: two case studies of Gujarati women

## Introduction

This chapter focuses on the pregnancy and childbirth experiences of the Gujarati women within the same household who were related to each other by marriage and were both expecting their first baby about the same time. From the accounts given by the Gujarati women in the preceding chapters, it is evident that their husbands' female relatives exercised considerable influence in the management of pregnancy and postnatal care. The differences in opinion about appropriate care and behaviour during pregnancy emerged as a major source of tension and conflict between the women and their female relatives. These issues are examined in some length to assess the possible impact of the two different approaches to managing childbirth and the strategy that the daughters-in-law used to negotiate their passage through pregnancy and childbirth.

The accounts of daughters-in-law are based on separate interviews conducted during pregnancy and six weeks after childbirth, and include analyses of comments and interactions between daughters-in-law and mothers-in-law. Although the level of emotional and practical support provided by the women's own parents is not insignificant, particularly in the postnatal period, the discussion is confined to the women's interactions with their husbands' relatives, reflecting the fact that they spent the greater proportion of their time with their husbands' family.

One of the important features of the South Asian household is that it is complex and defies simple definition. This heterogeneity is reflected in the considerable variation in the formation and composition of families both in the case studies and in the rest of the book. Although the structure and composition of South Asian families has been in a process of transition, extended families are still common. A generalized version of extended households has been described as households containing more than two generations, commonly elderly parent/s, married sons and their wives and children and/or unmarried sons and daughters living under one roof, but not necessarily sharing financial resources or functioning as a single unit. However, family formulations are extremely varied. Ahmad (1996a: 54) points out that such families are universal neither in Britain nor in South Asia and cites the explanation provided by Anwar (1979: 52) to suggest that any extra-familial kin who maintain a relationship of some intimacy with members of a nuclear family can be understood as extended family.

The structure of South Asian families has been affected by many different factors: immigration; the changes in marriage patterns, including the increase in the number of ethnically mixed marriages; occupational mobility; and the greater participation of women in the labour market which has also influenced power relationships within the family (Westwood and Bhachu 1988; Stopes-Roe and Cochrane 1990).

From my observation and discussions with the women it became apparent that women who lived in an extended family found that their behaviour was closely scrutinized and regulated by rules and codes set by older members of the family. Among the women there was a definite pecking order, with the mother-in-law occupying the place at the top of the female hierarchy. The younger women in these families were obliged to maintain the family's honour by regulating their behaviour and observing family customs and traditions. Evidence suggests that, in Britain, the older members of the family sometimes perceive the indigenous cultural values and language as a threat to their own cultural identity (Westwood and Bhachu 1988; Stopes-Roe and Cochrane 1990; Ahmad 1996a). In addition, my observation of the Gujarati families suggested that some older women also perceive the acquisition of education and economic independence by younger female members of the family as a challenge to their authority and status. Thus the only possible course of action open to these older members of the family was to impose traditional beliefs and values on the younger members of the family in a way which allowed them to retain some of their influence and status.

Before examining the women's experiences of pregnancy and childbirth, it is important to understand the structure of the two families and the nature of relationships within extended households.

Within the South Asian community, kinship ties between individual members of a family are vested with considerable significance. They not only provide an instant method of identifying the branch of the family from which the relationship stems, but the use of precise terminology in the form of the suffix (signifying the precise relationship) attached to the first name of the individual serves a dual function (Trivedi 1920). The formal recognition of kinship ties also provides a mechanism for preserving physical and social boundaries between members of the opposite sex within extended households. Since the discussion of women's experiences of childbirth is confined to the interactions between the women and their husband's relatives, the following terminology refers to women's relationships to various members of the husband's family:

*Sasra* – father-in-law
*Sasu* – mother-in-law
*Jeth* – husband's elder brother
*Jethani* – husband's elder brother's wife
*Dher* – husband's younger brother
*Dherani* – husband's younger brother's wife
*Narand* – husband's sister

## Case study of family A

The daughters-in-law in the two case studies have been given fictitious names to protect their identities and that of their family. In the first extended household, Meera (*Jethani*) and Lata (*Dherani*) were married to two brothers in the same family. They were both in their middle twenties; both had had secondary education and were in full-time employment at the time of their first interviews. Meera and Lata had been married within a year of each other. Meera (*Jethani*) became pregnant first. Meera and Lata lived in two separate self-contained flats which were separated by a flight of stairs. Meera and her husband owned the downstairs flat while Lata and her husband owned the top flat. To all intents and purposes the two flats were run as two independent households. Meera and Lata's parents-in-law, who also lived with them, moved freely between the two flats and treated the two separate flats as a joint household and controlled the family affairs and the lives of Lata and Meera. The husbands' married sisters who lived locally were also influential in family affairs and particularly in decisions involving their brothers' wives.

Meera's parents and other members of her family lived locally. Lata's parents lived abroad and her nearest relative in this country was her married brother who lived some distance away.

## Case study of family B

In the second extended household the two daughters-in-law, Geeta and Kamla, were married to two brothers in the same family and were expecting their first baby within six weeks of each other. Kamla and Geeta were in their late twenties, had completed secondary school education and had worked full-time before their pregnancies. Geeta (*Jethani*) was from a different Gujarati caste and was married to the older brother. It was Geeta's second marriage after her first marriage had ended in divorce. Geeta and her husband lived in a joint household with her widowed mother-in-law and her husband's older unmarried sister (*Narand*). Kamla (*Dherani*) was married to the younger brother and they lived apart from the rest of the family in their own flat but in the same neighbourhood.

Kamla's parents and other members of her family lived in the neighbourhood. Geeta's parents lived in India and her nearest relatives in Britain were her uncle and aunt who were both doctors.

Since the structure and composition of the two families were slightly different, it is important to give a brief history about the family relationships that existed between the daughters-in-law and the family. Although what the family members expected from the daughters-in-law in both families was culturally similar, in one family Geeta's pregnancy and her behaviour became a focal point for expressing discontent within the family. This was particularly significant in the case of Geeta and her in-laws because Geeta's first marriage had ended in divorce; also her status within her second husband's family was undermined by the fact that she was from a different Gujarati caste. Although inter-caste marriages have become more acceptable generally, Geeta still encountered difficulties gaining acceptance in her husband's family because her previous marriage had been unsuccessful. While Geeta was striving to establish her status in her husband's family, the recent death of her father-in-law had left her mother-in-law and older unmarried sister-in-law feeling less secure about their position within the household. As will become evident, in the struggle to establish a new pecking order Geeta's pregnancy became a battleground for expressing resentment and asserting influence.

While Geeta was constantly affected by the presence of her in-laws, Kamla, who lived apart from her in-laws, was not. Kamla and her husband belonged to the same caste and their marriage had been arranged by their families. The fact that Kamla's parents lived in the neighbourhood also placed her in a stronger position to manage her relationship with her husband's relatives.

As previously stated, the main areas over which the extended family had influence were on women's behaviour in relation to their pregnancy, decisions concerning the management of care during pregnancy, decisions involving preparation for birth and the management of postnatal care. Each of these themes will be explored to identify similarities and differences in their approach to negotiating care and the strategy they used to circumvent restrictions imposed by their female relatives.

## Attitudes to pregnancy

Although the four women in the two families were expecting their first babies, their accounts suggested that not all of them were excited about the prospect of having a baby. Considering the tremendous social pressure for women to bear children and the fact that they were expecting their first babies, this ambiguity was particularly striking. For instance, of the four women, Meera and Lata's strong reservations about their pregnancies appeared incongruous with their relatives' aspirations. The fundamental differences in attitudes concerning the appropriate status of the women and their biological destiny seemed to lie at the core of the apparent disagreements between the women and their husbands' relatives. In the case of Lata and Meera their pregnancies became very much a family affair as soon as the pregnancies were confirmed. The news of Meera and Lata's pregnancies was greeted with a great deal of approval by their husbands' relatives. It was evident that for the women's in-laws their pregnancy signalled their willingness to conform so as to make their behaviour appropriate to their role:

> I was shocked to learn that I was pregnant because we had not planned to have a baby just yet as we had been married for only two years. I prayed for the pregnancy test to be negative. I was very upset at first because I was not emotionally prepared. As far as my in-laws are concerned a woman is not supposed to worry about a career . . . they have very orthodox views and they believe that a woman's place is to be in the home and have children. For me my job is very important and not just for financial reasons.
>
> (Meera)

It is evident that Meera and Lata's attitudes towards pregnancy and motherhood were informed by priorities which conflicted with those of their in-laws. Meera and Lata's attitudes in many respects appeared closely aligned with the notion of planned parenthood and ideas supporting the emancipation of women which offered a greater choice and freedom to move beyond the traditionally prescribed role of a wife, mother and housekeeper. For the older generation of South Asian women who were brought up with different expectations, such attitudes represented a challenge to cultural traditions which they respected and wished to perpetuate into the next generation. It is not surprising to find that the concerns Meera and Lata expressed about the likely impact of their unplanned pregnancies on their employment and career opportunities met with little sympathy:

> We have very recently bought our flat so pregnancy was the last thing on our mind . . . I can't afford to give up my job. My *Sasu* [mother-in-law] used to remind my husband that we were married over three years and yet there was no sign of a baby. They [parents-in-law] had started to suspect that there was something wrong with us. When she [mother-in-law] found out about my pregnancy she gave a sigh of relief!
>
> (Lata)

In contrast, Geeta and Kamla, who were also part of an extended household, were happy to be pregnant, as both of them had been trying to conceive for some time. However, the news of their pregnancies aroused different responses from their husbands' relatives. For example, Kamla reported that members of her husband's family were delighted when she announced her pregnancy:

> My *Sasu* [mother-in-law] is especially pleased because my father-in-law passed away recently. It has given her hope. She [mother-in-law] and I weren't that close before but since I have become pregnant she has shown interest in my health and also offered to help. My *Narand* [husband's sisters] are also pleased to become aunts for the first time . . .
>
> (Kamla)

Kamla explained that considering the circumstances she felt that she had forfeited the right to expect support from her husband's relatives because she had ignored her mother-in-law's earlier entreaties to have a baby and also because she had chosen to set up her own home away from the extended family. However, far from being distant and disinterested, she was overwhelmed by the amount of goodwill and interest shown towards her pregnancy by her husband's relatives.

Geeta, on the other hand, who lived with her husband's family, placed a totally different interpretation on her mother-in-law's attitude towards her pregnancy. For example, Geeta spoke at great length about her own parents' positive reactions to her pregnancy. However, unlike Kamla, she did not acknowledge her mother-in-law's interest in her pregnancy although her mother-in-law was present throughout the interview: 'As soon as my pregnancy was confirmed I phoned my parents in India. They are over the moon. If my parents were around they would have spoilt me – they would have lavished me with care and attention' (Geeta).

Geeta's apparent refusal to acknowledge her mother-in-law's pleasure in her pregnancy and her other comments concerning her mother-in-law's attitude towards her pregnancy were weak attempts to disguise the conflict which existed in the family. The poor relationship between Geeta and her husband's relatives made a major impact on Geeta's perception of her pregnancy and the way she transacted care during pregnancy and after childbirth. For example, although Geeta's mother-in-law was the first person to recognize the symptoms of her pregnancy, she was not prepared to accept that her mother-in-law's intuitive knowledge was superior to that of her aunt who was a doctor:

> She [mother-in-law] was the first person to notice that I was pregnant because I had dizzy spells and morning sickness. I couldn't believe that she [mother-in-law] was right when my aunt who is a qualified doctor did not think I was pregnant and the tests done by my doctor were also negative.

## Negotiating care and support during pregnancy

Although the women's experiences of managing care during pregnancy within extended households were not unlike those reported by other Gujarati women, the examination of the same issues from the perspectives of two women within the same household provides an insight into the strategy they used in negotiating care. The issues highlighted by the mismatch in expectations of the role of daughters-in-law and the differences in attitudes towards pregnancy and motherhood continued to have a major impact on the decisions the women took to negotiate care and support in pregnancy.

Further differences in attitudes towards pregnancy were also evident in the way the women and their mothers-in-law regarded pregnancy. For example, from the interactions which took place between the women and their mothers-in-law, it was apparent that they had different views on the care and treatment of pregnant women. While Geeta's mother-in-law believed that pregnancy was a natural occurrence and it was not unusual for women to experience a certain amount of discomfort or ailments, Geeta disagreed:

> My aunt suggested that I should take plenty of rest and my doctor prescribed some medicine for the sickness and the bleeding. My mother-in-law did not think it was necessary for me to stay in a bed all day because she felt that sickness and slight bleeding is common in early pregnancy. They [older women] used to work quite a lot in their pregnancies and she [mother-in-law] expected me to help with the household chores and felt I was making too much fuss about my pregnancy.

When Geeta's mother-in-law was invited to give her view about how pregnant women should be cared for, she remarked: 'I had four children and women in my time did not take to bed. I spoke to women in the temple and they also said the same thing. In our time, we believed that it was important to keep active . . . if you speak to other women they will say the same.'

Meera and Lata also reported similar disagreements concerning their mother-in-law's expectations of how they should conduct themselves during pregnancy and the level of support and care they should expect from the family:

> My mother-in-law is not pleased with me at the moment because I complained that I'm getting very tired. My mother-in-law thinks that I am making too much fuss because she had eight children and she never made any fuss. My mother-in-law forgets that she did not go out to work and besides in Africa she had servants to do all the housework. My mother-in-law believes that an office job is not demanding and she also does not understand why I have to work outside the home.
>
> (Lata)

Although older women's experiences of pregnancy and motherhood were managed under different circumstances, it is evident that they were expecting their daughters-in-law to conduct themselves as they had done and were not prepared to make allowances for daughters-in-law who continued working during their pregnancies. There is evidence to suggest that the increasing participation of South Asian women in waged work has had a significant impact on the dynamics of family relationships as the traditional division of labour and hierarchies within the household are being challenged (Westwood and Bhachu 1988).

It was evident that the difficult family relationships exacerbated the physical and emotional stress the women experienced during pregnancy. While Meera was able to rely on her parents, who lived in the neighbourhood, to sustain her during this stressful period, Lata was in a less fortunate position and had fewer opportunities to get away from her in-laws as her parents lived abroad. Her only source of support in this country was her brother with whom she was allowed limited contact:

> Unfortunately, my mother is too far to give me support. My mum lives in Kenya and I don't have any support or a place I can go to, to get a break from my in-laws. I have a brother in the East End but my parents-in-law do not like me to visit him because they [parents-in-law] believe that it is a rough area.

From the comments made by Meera and Lata it was evident that they were both struggling to free themselves of the constraints imposed by their parents-in-law. While the close proximity of the two households enabled their parents-in-law to keep a close watch on their behaviour during their pregnancies, united by their opposition of their parents-in-law Meera and Lata were able to draw strength from each other. For Lata this support was vital to survive in an extended family as, unlike Meera, she did not have any close relatives in the neighbourhood to provide support during this difficult time: 'The only person I can talk to freely is Meera because we both have to put up with our parents-in-law. It has also been helpful to talk to Meera about my pregnancy because she just had a baby.'

Of the four women in the case studies, Kamla appeared to be best placed to enjoy support from both sides of her family. However, she was aware that if she was still living with her mother-in-law she would not have been able to avoid the conflict which Geeta had experienced: 'In the beginning I felt constantly tired so I used to go to sleep as soon as I returned home from work. I don't think I would have been so free to do as I please. Although they [husband's relations] would tell you to rest you would still feel obliged to help.'

Although the intricacies of managing relationships within extended households is difficult enough at the best of times, from the women's accounts it is evident that during pregnancy they acquired an added dimension. For example, a mismatch in expectations about the appropriate level of care and support provided and received was also evident in Geeta's account:

> I suffered from sickness and extreme tiredness for nearly four months. My *Fai* [father's sister] advised me to stay in bed. My *Fai* is a doctor so I value her advice but my mother-in-law expected me to help her with the household chores. The midwife at the clinic also suggested that my husband should bring tea for me in bed before I got up. My mother-in-law would not allow my husband to prepare breakfast for me because she did not consider it proper for a man to make breakfast for his wife. My mother-in-law has old fashioned views – she told me that pregnant

women in her times did not take to bed with minor complaints in pregnancy.

It was evident that dietary advice or dietary restrictions, advice about health in pregnancy and ceremonial rituals were important aspects of the traditional method of managing care in pregnancy. Given that in extended households women's conduct during pregnancy is under constant scrutiny, any decisions women make about these practices require delicate negotiation. For instance, although neither Meera nor Lata openly questioned the merit of traditional practices, they found ways of minimizing their impact or ignoring them:

> At home I am a vegetarian because my in-laws are very orthodox and would not like their daughters-in-law to eat eggs or meat. When I go out with my husband I eat meat but only chicken, no red meat. Once my in-laws confronted me and said that someone had seen me eating meat but I just denied it. There is nothing they can do when I am out.
>
> (Lata)

The fact that such instructions were given in the presence of their husbands to ensure that they were strictly observed did not prevent Meera and Lata from finding ways of getting around the restrictions:

> As soon as I told my mother-in-law that I was pregnant she told me that there are certain things I cannot do while I am pregnant and one of them was a ban on eating bananas and sesame seeds. I have to agree and follow her instructions otherwise she would complain about me to my husband. I agree to most things and then I do as I please when she is not around.
>
> (Lata)

As previously indicated, in addition to dietary restrictions, observation of ceremonial rituals was an important element of securing transition through pregnancy. The older women in the family retained their faith in the ceremonial rituals as a means of safeguarding the pregnancy and therefore wished to perpetuate the family traditions. However, the younger generation of women like Meera and Lata found it difficult to believe that they served any useful purpose as no explanations were given:

> I have not washed my hair for the past seven months. My mother-in-law told me that pregnant women in our family are not allowed to wash their hair. I would have found it a lot easier to accept if she had given an explanation for it. Since my in-laws live with us it is not easy to ignore the rules they lay down for us. It was a real nuisance while I was working because I was worried about attracting bad comments from my colleagues at work.
>
> (Meera)

When Lata realized the difficulties Meera had in observing the hair washing restriction, she decided to use the information she had gained to her advantage in order to lessen the impact of the restriction during her pregnancy. When Lata became suspicious that she might be pregnant she spoke to Meera first to find a way around this problem:

> I first heard about the hair washing restriction when Meera became pregnant. As I knew that this restriction would also apply to me as soon as my pregnancy was confirmed, I went to the hairdresser first to have a hair cut so that it would be easier to manage. When my mother-in-law realized I was pregnant she told me that from that day I was not to wash my hair and she told me in the presence of my husband to make sure that I did not ignore her instructions. I think it is unhygienic. I was really upset because I was working and I didn't want to go to work looking a mess.
>
> (Lata)

Many older women, of Meera and Lata's mother-in-law's generation, had their children under different circumstances in countries in East Africa where Asian women rarely engaged in waged work and where traditional childbirth practices predominated. Since the rituals and restrictions did not require women to cross cultural boundaries, observation of such restrictions was not perceived by older women to be problematic. It was not surprising that older women expected younger women under their jurisdiction to follow suit, and any attempt to reject practices which had served them well in their own times was incomprehensible: 'My mother-in-law told me that she didn't have any problem looking after her hair through her pregnancies but then she didn't go out to work whereas I do and personal appearance does count' (Meera).

Meera and Lata also believed that older women in East Africa lived among their own communities which shared similar beliefs and values and were, unlike them, rarely exposed to people from different cultures who might have questioned their beliefs. Both women felt that such restrictions were outdated and meaningless impositions on their lives but felt obliged to keep up with family traditions because they were concerned to preserve their *izzat* or reputation in the community: 'In the end I did accept it because it would have caused too much upset in the family. I used to use dry shampoo and damp towel to clean my scalp. My mother-in-law used to disapprove of that as well because I was breaking the tradition' (Lata).

Raja's (1993) investigation of intergenerational differences in attitudes towards the concept of health and illness within the Gujarati Hindu community reports similar findings.

It is evident that Meera and Lata tried to accommodate their mother-in-law's wishes, as they were reticent about publicly defying their mother-in-law's authority. In the case of Geeta and Kamla the situation was more complicated. Kamla had lived apart from her husband's family and the distance of time and space had allowed her to negotiate her relationship with members of her husband's family on her own terms. Consequently the ties of obligation towards her in-laws did not carry the weight they had done previously. The sense of independence gave Kamla courage to make her own decision during pregnancy and to reject any advice of her mother-in-law if it did not suit her: 'I have changed my diet to suit myself. My mother-in-law has not given me any advice about diet but she tells Geeta what she should eat and what foods she should avoid. My mother-in-law does not live with me so she does not know what I eat.'

Kamla maintained her independent stance in all matters concerning the management of her pregnancy including the observation of ceremonial rituals:

> Once my mother-in-law learnt that I was pregnant she told me that I should not wash my hair until after I had the *Khoro* [lap] ceremony at the seventh month. I told her that I had to wash my hair because I was working. Yet my mother-in-law and other people who strongly believe in such things are not prepared to accept that I have to look good for my job. My mother-in-law told me it was up to me, as she was not going to force me. I was made to feel like an outcast and a naughty person to disobey.

Kamla had declined to observe the ritual at the beginning of her pregnancy, as she excused herself from taking part in any further ceremonies. She also had her husband's backing to withstand her mother-in-law's exhortation:

> Since the *Khoro* ceremony involves washing hair for the first time, my husband and I felt that it was pointless for me to undergo this ceremony because I had been washing my hair regularly. My mother-in-law still insisted that I should have a *Khoro*. She was really upset and felt that I had let her down. I felt that since Geeta was observing everything, my mother-in-law would not be deprived of her pleasure.

In contrast, Geeta's attitude towards traditional childbirth practices was more ambiguous. Her inconsistent approach to negotiating care during pregnancy was apparent from her selective rejection and acceptance of restrictions and rituals (see also Drury 1991). For example, any dietary advice given by Geeta's mother-in-law was contradicted and rejected if it did not accord with advice given by her aunt:

> *Geeta*: I have increased my appetite a lot – I am always hungry. I like eating hot spicy foods and especially things made out of rice. My mother-in-law feels I am eating too much rice. She told me to stop eating rice and bananas.
>
> *Mother-in-law*: Rice is not good because it does not contain much goodness and it also makes you fat.
>
> *Geeta*: I don't believe in any of these restrictions. I love banana and rice. I didn't eat them for a while and then I asked my aunt who told me that no harm will come to me if I eat anything I enjoyed eating so I eat everything and ignore my mother-in-law.

*Mother-in-law*: Even the doctor advises you to cut down starchy foods like rice.

On the other hand, Geeta did not have any objections to observing an injunction on hair washing during pregnancy and participating in the ceremonial ritual of *Khoro*. Given that many aspects of Geeta's pregnancy became foci for confrontations it was remarkable that, when it came to observing ceremonial rituals, Geeta did not put up any resistance. It was more remarkable that Geeta did not take advantage of the precedent set up by Kamla who had refused to observe any ceremonial rituals:

> My mother-in-law had told me before I became pregnant that I would not be allowed to wash my hair for the first seven months of pregnancy. My mother-in-law had also told Kamla who became pregnant before me but Kamla refused to listen to my mother-in-law's instructions. I didn't want to upset my mother-in-law and also in case something did go wrong with the baby – she would always remind me that I had been disrespectful to our family deity.

When Geeta's mother-in-law was invited to give her views on the significance of rituals and restrictions she remarked:

> I have done my duty to my daughters-in-law. I have explained to Geeta and Kamla how important it is that they should watch what they eat and the care they should take to have a safe delivery . . . all women in our family have followed these traditions for generations. If now they go against my wishes then it is up to them.

It is evident that for the older generation of women, the rejection of traditions represented a threat to their social order as the observation of rituals provided a mechanism for social exchange. It is not surprising that the stance adopted by Kamla was perceived as a threat on the basis that once one cultural rule was broken, it introduced weakness in the system which would have far-reaching consequences for the future.

## Antenatal preparation

For older Asian women who had their children in East Africa or in the Indian subcontinent formal antenatal preparation involving attendance at classes was an alien concept. Although older women in their time may not have had any formal training to prepare for birth, the enactment of ceremonial rituals such as the *Khoro* prepared the pregnant women for childbirth. In addition to preparation involving rituals, physical preparation for birth included the taking of herbal preparations to speed the birth process. With the exception of Kamla, for Meera, Lata and Geeta who were living in an extended household, antenatal preparation included both the traditional form involving their participation in the ceremonial rituals and the classes offered by the maternity services.

Although older female relatives exercised a great deal of influence over many aspects of pregnancy, on the whole their jurisdiction did not extend beyond the boundary of the home. Geeta, however, claimed that her mother-in-law disapproved of her son attending classes or assisting his wife in labour:

> She [mother-in-law] thinks it is shameful to have the presence of any man during childbirth. I don't agree . . . why not? I have told my husband that I can't cope without his support. My mother-in-law did not like it when my husband attended classes with me but there is nothing she can do about it.

Meera and Lata, on the other hand, reported that their mother-in-law did not object to their attending parentcraft classes provided that they kept away from labour and postnatal wards. As was explained earlier in Chapter 5, many Asian women believe that parturient women are agents of pollution and other pregnant women are advised to keep away from them to avoid any mishaps:

> My mother-in-law does not know that I have already made a tour of the labour ward with the other pregnant women in my class. When my *Narand* [sister-in-law] informed my mother-in-law about the labour ward visit, she [mother-in-law] told me that she wouldn't like me to go. I didn't want to upset her [mother-in-law] so I didn't tell her that I had already done so.
>
> (Meera)

In Meera's case, lack of prior knowledge about the labour ward visit had prevented her mother-in-law from taking appropriate action, but in Lata's case, her mother-in-law left her with little doubt about the importance she attached to this injunction:

> I knew that my mother-in-law would not like me to go anywhere near the labour ward because when Meera had her baby I wasn't allowed to visit her in the hospital or allowed to go near her for the next six weeks. When I asked my mother-in-law for an explanation she told me that Meera was in an 'unclean' state. My husband and I were desperate to see Meera's new baby so we paid a secret visit to Meera at her mum's house.

Once the rule was broken, Lata claimed that she lost all her inhibition about touring the labour ward and she did not have any hesitation in holding a newborn baby. Lata, however, was very anxious to explain her reasons for going against the wishes of her mother-in-law: 'It is not that I don't believe in our culture or that I want to disobey my in-laws. It is just that I don't believe that any harm could come to me or my baby . . . I will just have to wait and see when the baby comes!'

Geeta and Kamla had also ignored the advice of their mother-in-law and visited the labour ward during their pregnancies. However, Kamla reported that when she was convalescing in the postnatal ward, Geeta obeyed the instruction of their mother-in-law and kept away:

> When I was in the postnatal ward everyone from both sides of the family visited me except Geeta because she was pregnant. Geeta and I did not believe that any harm would come to her. Anyway . . . she [Geeta] was not prepared to upset my mother-in-law so she used to wait in the car while other members of the family visited me.

The experiences of Meera, Lata and Geeta suggest that relationships within extended households are based on adjustment and readjustment and recognition of norms or boundaries within which relationships are negotiated. This is evident from the fact that neither Meera, Lata nor, to some extent, Geeta was prepared to defy their in-laws openly, but on the other hand they were prepared to extend the boundaries when they thought it was to their advantage. For example, they were able to participate fully in the parentcraft classes, although aware of the potential risk of causing family friction. They were prepared to take a chance in the knowledge that their mother-in-law's influence was curtailed by her lack of familiarity with western childbirth practices.

## Postnatal support within extended households

Since it was traditional practice among many Gujarati women to return to their parental home after childbirth, their postnatal experience was determined by who provided the support to them after childbirth. After Meera and Kamla were discharged from the postnatal ward, they went straight to their parents' homes and stayed there for the '40 days' convalescence period. Since Lata and Geeta did not have close relatives in the neighbourhood, they returned home to their mother-in-laws' care. In the case of Meera and Lata there appeared to be very little difference in the quality of practical help they received from their families. When Lata returned from the hospital she found the practical support provided by her mother-in-law was most helpful:

> My mother-in-law has been very helpful. She did all the housework and cooking when I came home. She has been very good to me and while I was in the hospital she used to smuggle food into the ward because I didn't like the hospital food. She did not want me to do anything except attend to the baby's needs.

Meera had also enjoyed the same care and attention at her mother's house:

> When I was discharged from the hospital, my parents came to fetch me from the hospital. I have been staying here for the past five weeks. While I am staying with my parents I have had lots of rest, help and guidance from my mum. I have found it more comfortable to be with

> my mother. I do not have to watch what I do or say, and I feel at ease to ask and receive help. They do practically everything for the baby and I only have to feed him.

However, in the postnatal interview there was a remarkable change in the attitude of Lata towards her mother-in-law. She was not only grateful to her mother-in-law but also expressed remorse for defying her mother-in-law by visiting the labour ward during her pregnancy against her mother-in-law's wishes:

> She [daughter] was born underweight. I feel it is perhaps because I had disobeyed my mother-in-law during my pregnancy. I had visited Meera after she gave birth and had also visited the labour ward against my mother-in-law's advice. I do feel guilty. I can't put these thoughts out of my mind. I can't tell anyone . . . not even my husband why I am so upset. Perhaps I should have listened to my mother-in-law's advice.

Pillsbury (1978) notes similar regrets on the part of professional Chinese women regarding lack of observance of the Chinese practice of 'doing the month'.

In many respects the level of support Kamla and Geeta received in the postnatal period was similar to that of Meera and Lata. However, in the case of Geeta, her experience was affected by the tension which had existed between her and her in-laws during her pregnancy. Geeta appeared to be more restrained during the postnatal interview, which took place in the presence of her husband's older sister, but she did not hide her feelings. The disagreement about dietary advice resurfaced:

> I had the traditional foods which my mother-in-law prepared for me for a few days but when I asked the midwife whether I should carry on eating this special diet, she advised me that it is better to eat ordinary food. My mother-in-law felt that I should carry on eating the special diet for a few more days. My mother-in-law believes that this special diet helps with backache and recovery especially as she had done it after each of her pregnancies. After I consulted the midwife I told my mother-in-law to stop preparing special foods for me.

Geeta's accounts seemed to be giving contradictory messages, as the comments she made earlier suggested that she was happy to receive traditional food prepared by her mother-in-law:

> When I was in hospital my mother-in-law used to bring traditional foods for me because the hospital meals were inadequate and were nothing like the traditional foods recommended for women after childbirth. I used to share the food my mother-in-law brought with other Indian women in my ward.

## Summary

The experiences of the women in extended households provide an interesting insight into the dynamics of family relationships and the process of negotiating care during pregnancy and childbirth, suggesting that this process is far more complex than it would seem. It is evident that the stresses and strains of maintaining hierarchical relationships were exacerbated by the competing demands of the traditional and medical models of childbirth which the women were required to satisfy.

However, the accounts of the women also suggest that once their pregnancy was over and they were back in the folds of their community and no longer having to adapt their behaviour and attitudes to suit the demands of a 'hospital birth package', the conflicts between the women and their in-laws rapidly melted away.

## Annotated bibliography

Ahmad, W.I.U. (1996a) 'Family obligations and social change among Asian communities', in W.I.U. Ahmad and K. Atkin (eds) *'Race' and Community Care.* Buckingham: Open University Press.

This paper explores ideas about social obligations and social support networks and their importance in the social and economic survival and success of South Asian communities. The discussion focuses on various factors such as the nature of family structure and history, personal and moral identity, class and gender, which influence the negotiation of obligation. The discussion also considers the meanings and values such a tradition has in the present time.

Drury, B. (1991) Sikh girls and the maintenance of an ethnic culture, *New Community*, 17(3): 387–99.

This paper examines the extent to which certain aspects of Sikh cultural and religious values have been retained by young Sikh women who formed a part of the second generation of women who were either born in Britain or had arrived in Britain under the age of 5. The author analyses gender differences and the extent to which external and internal pressures were factors in the women's decision to retain or abandon cultural and religious traditions.

Westwood, S. and Bhachu, P. (1988) (eds) *Enterprising Women: Economy and Gender Relations*. London: Routledge.

This book contains a series of papers on ethnic minority women's involvement in paid work and its consequences on family and gender relationships. Papers by Westwood, Bhachu and Warrier provide an insight into how Asian women balance the competing demands of being workers, wives and mothers.

# 8

# Conclusion

The main objective of this book has been to provide an insight into the experiences of childbirth from the perspectives of two different groups of South Asian women in Britain with a particular focus on the way they negotiated care between medical and traditional childbirth practices. In bringing this book to a close, I would like to summarize some of the main issues raised by the women and place them within the context of the wider theoretical debate concerning control in childbirth.

Preceding chapters have argued that any analysis of South Asian women's experiences of pregnancy and childbirth must proceed on a number of levels, if it is to avoid some of the pitfalls of previous research. This is important for several reasons. First, any discussion of South Asian women's experiences of childbirth must be placed within the wider context of race, ethnicity and racism to appreciate not only how these factors impinge on the lives of South Asians but also to acknowledge the tremendous diversity which exists within the British South Asian communities. Second, South Asian women do not live in a cultural vacuum: they are affected by childbirth practices in both their own and the indigenous culture. And last but not least, it is necessary to draw parallels between the views and experiences of South Asian and British women to ensure that the perspectives of South Asian women are neither overlooked nor marginalized.

While it is misleading to make broad generalizations based on a relatively small sample, the Gujarati and Bangladeshi women consulted during the course of the study raise important questions both for women generally and for those involved in providing maternity care.

One of the most important points to emerge from the accounts of Gujarati and Bangladeshi women was that, although there were individual variations, their range of experiences of childbirth strongly reflected the differences in cultural, religious, economic and migration histories. There can be no justification for treating women from South Asian communities as if they are all the same. These differences in experiences were further reflected in the women's attitudes towards conception and their responses to medical and traditional models of managing care during pregnancy and childbirth. An underlying concern was the question of choice or control the women exercised in influencing decisions on the management of pregnancy, intra-partum and post-partum care.

From the discussion in Chapters 2 and 3, it was evident that the women's attitudes towards pregnancy and motherhood were affected by the wider social location of women. These were manifest in the social construction of motherhood and the expectation of the women's role in childbearing, the strong disapproval of women who are infertile and of conception occurring outside marriage. These cultural values were shared by both groups of women. However, a clear departure from some of these values was more evident among the Gujarati than the Bangladeshi women. It was apparent that many Gujarati women were beginning to see themselves as career women rather than solely in the traditional role of wives and mothers. This change in values naturally led to conflict and the need to devise strategies to negotiate the move away from traditional values.

Women who were unable to negotiate this transition were generally more dissatisfied with their lack of control over, for example, family spacing or the choice of whether or not to pursue a career. Moreover, the circumstances under which the women became pregnant depended not only on their cultural and religious attitudes to birth control but also on who had the responsibility for taking precautions to prevent a pregnancy. The lack of shared responsibility for preventing an unwanted pregnancy was often more problematic for Gujarati women and, in some cases, produced a strong reaction against an unwanted pregnancy.

Moving on to issues affecting the management of care during pregnancy, intra-partum and postnatal care, the accounts of women in Chapters 4, 5 and 6 suggest that some aspects of traditional childbirth practices were shared by both groups of women. The women's ability to exercise control over decisions affecting the management of pregnancy was determined by how much they were influenced by the medical management of pregnancy and how much by the traditional management of pregnancy supervised by their female relatives. While traditional female-centred management of pregnancy placed greater emphasis on particular diets, remedies and rituals to enable women to make a safe transition from pregnancy to motherhood, medical management of pregnancy required confirmation of pregnancy by their doctor, and attendance at antenatal clinics for routine tests and examination, antenatal education and dietary and health advice given by the medical professionals.

For Gujarati women, the two very different approaches to the management of pregnancy created a great deal of conflict. This was partly due to the fact that many of them were fully conversant with the western medical system and were more open to persuasion to accept the medical model of care during pregnancy. At the same time, Gujarati women who were living in an extended household were expected to follow the advice given by their older female relatives. Those who faced this dilemma often, although not always, appeared anxious to reject the influence of the older female relatives, but they rarely questioned any aspects of medical care. However, the matter was more complex – the women neither adhered wholeheartedly to, nor entirely rejected, either approach.

The accounts of Gujarati women expecting their first baby suggested that they placed greater faith in western medicine and were very eager to seek medical confirmation of the pregnancy. They had a better record of attendance at the antenatal clinic and antenatal classes and took medical advice very seriously compared with those who had had previous experience of childbirth in Britain. This pattern of behaviour was continued by many first-time mothers right up to the time of delivery and the post-partum period.

Bangladeshi women, on the other hand, were not only anxious to observe purdah restrictions but also appear to have been guided by their previous knowledge of the traditional management of pregnancy. As a result, many Bangladeshi women did not worry unduly about obtaining medical confirmation of pregnancy nor did they consider it necessary to attend antenatal clinics early in pregnancy or attend antenatal classes. In fact, some women with previous experience of antenatal care in Britain deliberately delayed reporting their pregnancy to avoid attending clinics. Therefore, one could conclude that while Bangladeshi women were glad to receive medical care, they none the less determined how soon they availed themselves of it. Although they did not openly set out to defy medical control, their decision to delay seeking advice is none the less a form of resistance to medical control. It is, however, important to stress that the Bangladeshi women's reluctance to come forward for antenatal care was also due to reasons such as difficulties in gaining access to clinics, communication problems and the lack of childcare facilities.

The relative positions of the two groups of women and the significant others in their lives as regards childbirth determined the context for negotiating care. For example, Bangladeshi women were generally inclined towards traditional childbirth practices and, whenever possible, they made every effort to avoid medical childbirth practices. The position of Gujarati women, on the other hand, was ambiguous and complicated both by their greater familiarity with the western medical system and the need to take on board traditional practices favoured by their female relatives. Consequently, of the two communities, Gujarati women in some respects faced a greater challenge in negotiating care.

The way maternity care is organized and managed does not encourage women to take control of decisions affecting the management of their childbirth. The accounts of Gujarati and Bangladeshi women leave no doubt that both the social control of reproduction and the medicalization of childbirth implicitly and explicitly affected their decisions and behaviour concerning management of pregnancy, and intra-partum and post-partum care.

In many respects the worries of Gujarati and Bangladeshi women mirror those of white women, particularly with regard to the management of childbirth in hospital and the sense of powerlessness women feel when confronted with medical experts. Even if women succeed in resisting medical control of the management of their pregnancy, when it comes to choosing a place of delivery only the most well-informed and determined women can arrange to give birth at home instead of hospital. With almost 100 per cent hospitalization of birth, together with the increasing use of modern technology, most women find it difficult to resist medical control. Neither the Gujarati nor the Bangladeshi women appeared to put up any overt resistance to western medical practices. However, Bangladeshi women relied on their previous knowledge of childbirth to delay as long as possible their admission into hospital and thus minimize the control of obstetricians and medical technology. Bangladeshi women on the whole spent a shorter time in labour wards and had fewer medical interventions than Gujarati women.

When the current debate about control over childbirth is examined in the context of South Asian women in this study, a complex and contradictory picture emerges. On the one hand, this contradiction seems to be located in the issue of pollution and female-centred childbirth practices and, on the other hand, it is located in male-dominated medical practices. Ironically, it would appear that, because men in most traditional societies have a fear of contamination from pollution, they have been content to leave the responsibility of managing childbirth in the hands of women. At one level it would seem that the older women were colluding with the subjugation of women by perpetuating beliefs about pollution. At another level they were keeping the pollution belief alive to ensure that men were kept out of childbirth and also to safeguard their own status and influence within the family (Thompson 1985). Although ideas about pollution associated with parturient mothers may be construed as restrictive and outdated, it is important to note that many of the pollution rules are interwoven with strategies to allow women to recuperate and enjoy privileges in terms of food and enhanced status within the family. In an attempt to reject the pollution taboo and the influence of their female relatives many women, particularly Gujarati women, inadvertently ended up accepting western childbirth practices. Because of different patterns of immigration, most Bangladeshi women were not living in extended households and were therefore less likely to be subject to such pressures.

Although neither Bangladeshi nor Gujarati women appeared to be entirely satisfied with the treatment they had received from the medical professionals, their criticism was not directly linked to the lack of control over decisions affecting the management of pregnancy and childbirth. In fact, there was very little suggestion from either group of women that they objected to medicalization, hospitalization or a high-tech birth *per se* or that they equated such practices with a form of female oppression. While it is true that many women, particularly Bangladeshi women, expressed concern about receiving care from male health professionals and about difficulties in gaining access to health services because of language problems, they did not openly question either hospitalization or the medicalization of childbirth.

Such ambiguous attitudes on the part of South Asian women to western childbirth practices might lead one to conclude that South Asian women are less favourably inclined towards traditional childbirth practices than to the western medical model, and that they do not share the concerns of indigenous women regarding the lack of control over childbirth. Such conclusions represent only a superficial view. To understand fully the reasons why many women seemed to accept western childbirth practices with apparent equanimity, it is necessary to examine the women's attitudes in the broader context of institutionalized sexism and racism within the health service. It is an undeniable fact that, both at structural and organizational level, the National Health Service is dominated by men who wield a powerful influence over decisions affecting the management and delivery of health care. This influence is particularly evident with respect to the delivery of obstetric care (see, for instance, Oakley 1984). Another worrying aspect of the National Health Service which remains a major cause of concern for consumers within minority ethnic communities is the impact of institutionalized and individual racism affecting those, particularly women of childbearing age, who have the greatest need of health care services (Bowler 1993; Stubbs 1993).

In the present climate, when concern about the power of health professionals over women's bodies is a common topic for discussion, it is perhaps surprising to find that South Asian women are not expressing a similar concern. And yet in the early 1960s white women also believed that the doctors' judgement should not be questioned because their superior knowledge was based on specialist training. In fact, even women's organizations such as the National Childbirth Trust and the Association for Improvement in Maternity Services, which were set up to represent the interests of childbearing women, did not fully appreciate the danger of placing so much power in the hands of the medical profession.

Jenny Kitzinger (1990: 105), writing on the history of the National Childbirth Trust, points out that while the organization's main aim was to promote natural childbirth, the Trust took great pains to woo the medical profession. At the time, antenatal teachers trained by the National Childbirth Trust were instructed to encourage pregnant women to place their trust in the medical profession and to obey doctors' orders. The early campaigns of the Association for Improvement in Maternity Services were to demand hospital delivery for all women and pain-relieving drugs in labour to be made more freely available to all women. These demands were made with the best possible motives, and the implications of the lack of choice in the place of delivery and the disadvantages of pain-relieving drugs were only realized much later. In response to the dissatisfaction and alarm expressed by women about the lack of freedom to make their own decisions, both these organizations are now actively involved in campaigns to restore control over childbirth to women.

It would seem that the women who have gained most from the organizations, which have challenged medical authority, are predominantly white and middle class. The interests of working class women and women from black and minority ethnic communities have not been adequately addressed by these organizations. As a result, the information which enables white middle class women to take control over decisions affecting childbirth is not so readily accessible (see, for instance, NHS/CRD 1996). It is therefore not surprising to find that most women, including South Asian women, fail to question the authority of the medical profession. In addition, non-white women also experience racism (Rocheron *et al.* 1989; Bowler 1993).

For black and South Asian women who have been brought up under the shadow of western imperialism, it is difficult to challenge overt and covert racist attitudes which cast aspersions on minority ethnic peoples' beliefs and practices. Very often it is not only difficult to challenge covert racist attitudes but, worse still, there is tremendous pressure to internalize them. The most obvious examples of how racism affects South Asian women are demonstrated by the attitudes of Gujarati women towards both the medical profession and traditional childbirth practices. At one level South Asian women, in common with other British women, have to struggle with the sexist ideology which places health professionals on a pedestal. At another level, South Asian women have to cope with racist attitudes in British society. Very often the way to cope with the stress of racist attitudes is to internalize the racism, to accept the medical model and to reject traditional practices.

This position is not difficult to understand, given the historical tendency for the dominant culture, in this case British culture, to devalue any other beliefs. It was quite obvious from the women's accounts that they experienced the greatest pressure to reject their cultural ideology when they moved outside their community to obtain maternity care. Women were often worried about attracting derogatory comments from health professionals if they observed traditional diets or remedies or rituals. They were exposed to hostile comments from the nursing staff in the postnatal wards about traditional diets after childbirth.

As the argument presented in Chapter 2 suggests, traditional beliefs also come under assault from the numerous research projects specifically undertaken to unearth facts which are often used to explain the poor outcome of pregnancy among South Asians. There is also a tendency on the part of the health professionals to discredit the advisory role of anyone except those who receive medical training in the west. In this context, the literature makes the assumption that South Asian women, particularly older women, pose the greatest threat to medical authority because many of the traditional practices are promoted and supervised by older female relatives. Jordanova (1980: 51) suggests that male health professionals have often perceived traditional cures and ceremonies devised by women to restore health as a challenge to their more superior scientific knowledge. She asserts that the arguments used by male health professionals to dismiss such practices were based on sexist ideology which not only regarded women as amateur healers but also charged them with irresponsible behaviour for passing their knowledge to the next generation.

This book has, then, attempted to examine and understand how South Asian women living under the influence of two cultures make sense of their childbirth experiences. It has highlighted the fact that South Asian women, far from being homogeneous, are individuals with a wide range of ways of relating to pregnancy and coping with giving birth in Britain. Given that South Asian women who have recently settled in Britain face struggles on numerous fronts, it is not surprising that their fight against western childbirth practices does not take precedence over their efforts to adjust to life in a new country. Belonging to a different class and culture compounds their struggles. Furthermore, for a majority of South Asian women, the main struggle is to gain access to health services rather than question the sexual politics of reproduction within their own culture or in the white culture.

# References


Abdulla, T. and Zeidenstein, S. (1982) *Village Women of Bangladesh: Prospects for Change*. Oxford: Pergamon Press.

Abraham, R., Campbell-Brown, M., Haines, A.P., North, W.R.S., Hainsworth, V. and McFadyen, I.R. (1985) Diet during pregnancy in an Asian community in Britain – energy, protein, trace metals, fibres and minerals, *Human Nutrition: Applied Nutrition*, 39A: 23–35.

Adams, C. (1987) *Across Seven Seas and Thirteen Rivers*. London: THAP Books.

Ahmad, W.I.U., Kernohan, E.E.M. and Baker, M.R. (1989) Health of British Asians: a research review, *Community Medicine*, 11(1): 49–56.

Ahmad, W.I.U. (1992) The maligned healer: the 'hakim' and western medicine, *New Community*, 18(4): 521–36.

Ahmad, W.I.U. (ed.) (1993) Making black people sick: 'race', ideology and health research, in W.I.U. Ahmad (ed.) *'Race' and Health in Contemporary Britain*. Buckingham: Open University Press.

Ahmad, W.I.U. (1996a) Family obligations and social change among Asian communities, in W.I.U. Ahmad and K. Atkin (eds) *'Race' and Community Care*. Buckingham: Open University Press.

Ahmad, W.I.U. (1996b) Consanguinity and related demons: science and racism in the debate on consanguinity and birth outcome, in C. Samson and N. South (eds) *The Social Construction of Social Policy*. Basingstoke: Macmillan.

Ahmed, G. (1990) Family planning – religion and culture, *Maternity Action*, 43: 8–9.

Ahmed, G. and Watt, S. (1986) Understanding Asian women in pregnancy and confinement, *Midwives Chronicle and Nursing Notes*, 99(1180): 98–101.

Ahmet, L. (1990) A model for midwives – support for ethnic breastfeeding mothers, *Midwives Chronicle and Nursing Notes*, January: 5–7.

Anwar, M. (1979) *The Myth of Return: Pakistanis in Britain*. London: Heinemann.

Arms, S. (1975) *Immaculate Deception*. New York: Bantam Books.

Atkin, K., Ahmad, W.I.U. and Anionwu, E.N. (1998) Screening and counselling for sickle cell disorders and thalassaemia: the experiences of parents and health professionals, *Social Science and Medicine*, 47(11): 1639–51.

Aziz, K.M. and Maloney, C. (1985) *Life Stages, Gender and Fertility in Bangladesh*. Dhaka: Bangladesh International Centre for Diarrhoeal Disease Research.

Balarajan, R. and Botting, B. (1989) Perinatal mortality in England and Wales, variations by mother's country of birth (1982–85), *Health Trends*, 21: 79–84.
Balarajan, R. and Raleigh, V.S. (1990) Variations in perinatal, neonatal and postneonatal and infant mortality by mother's country of birth (1982–85), in M. Britton (ed.) *Mortality and Geography: A Review in the Mid-1980s, England and Wales*, Series DS, No. 9. London: HMSO.
Ballard, R. (1994) The emergence of Desh Pardesh, in R. Ballard (ed.) *Desh Pardesh: The South Asian Presence in Britain*. London: Hurst.
Barbour, R.S. (1990) Fathers: the emergence of a new consumer group, in J. Garcia, R. Kilpatrick and M. Richards (eds) *The Politics of Maternity Care: Services for Childbearing Women in Twentieth-Century Britain*. Oxford: Clarendon Press.
Barnes, R. (1982) Perinatal mortality and morbidity rates in Bradford, in I. McFadyen and J. MacVicar (eds) *Obstetric Problems of the Asian Community in Britain*. London: Royal College of Obstetricians and Gynaecologists.
Beard, P. (1982) Contraception in ethnic minority groups in Bedford, *Health Visitor*, 55(8): 417–19.
Bhachu, P. (1988) 'Apni Marzi Kardhi': home and work: Sikh women in Britain, in S. Westwood and P. Bhachu (1988) (eds) *Enterprising Women: Ethnicity, Economy and Gender Relations*. London: Routledge.
Bhopal, R.S. (1986) The inter-relationship of folk, traditional and western medicine within an Asian community in Britain, *Social Science and Medicine*, 22(1): 99–105.
Bhopal, R.S. (1992) Future research on the health of ethnic minorities: back to basics: a personal view, in W.I.U. Ahmad (ed.) *The Politics of 'Race' and Health*. Bradford: Race Relations Research Unit, University of Bradford, Bradford and Ilkley Community College.
Bhopal, R. and White, M. (1993) Health promotion for ethnic minorities: past, present and future, in W.I.U. Ahmad (ed.) *'Race' and Health in Contemporary Britain*. Buckingham: Open University Press.
Bhopal, R., Phillmore, P. and Kohli, H. (1991) Inappropriate use of the term 'Asian': an obstacle to ethnicity and health research, *Journal of Public Health Medicine*, 13(4): 244–46.
Birbalsingh, F. (1997) *From Pillar to Post: Indo-Caribbean Diaspora*. Toronto: TSAR.
Bissenden, J. (1979) The nutrition of the Asian immigrant mothers in relation to birthweight, *Proceedings of the Nutrition Society*, 38(3): 103A.
Blanchet, T. (1984) *Women, Pollution and Marginality: Meanings and Rituals of Birth in Rural Bangladesh*, Decca: The University Press Limited.
Bowler, I. (1993) 'They're not the same as us': midwives' stereotypes of South Asian descent maternity patients, *Sociology of Health and Illness*, 15(2): 157–78.
Brown, G.W. and Harris, T. (1978) *Social Origins of Depression*. London: Tavistock.
Bundey, S., Alam, H., Kaur, A., Mir, S. and Lancashire, R.J. (1989) Race, consanguinity and social features in Birmingham babies: a basis for prospective study, *Journal of Epidemiology and Community Health*, 44: 130–5.
Burghart, R. (ed.) (1987) *Hinduism in Great Britain: The Perpetuation of Religion in an Alien Cultural Milieu*. London: Tavistock.
Campbell, R. and Macfarlane, A. (1990) Recent debate on the place of birth, in J. Garcia, R. Kilpatrick and M. Richards (eds) *The Politics of Maternity Care: Services for Childbearing Women in Twentieth-Century Britain*. Oxford: Clarendon.

Caplan, P. (1985) *Class and Gender in India: Women and their Organisations in a South Indian City*. London: Tavistock.
Carey, S. and Skukur, A. (1985) A profile of the Bangladeshi in East London, *New Community*, 12(3): 405–17.
Cartwright, A. (1976) *How Many Children?* London: HMSO.
Cartwright, A. (1977) Mothers' experiences of induction, *British Medical Journal*, 17 September: 745–9.
Cartwright, A. (1979) *The Dignity of Labour?* London: Tavistock.
Charles, C. (1983) A midwife's experience of the Asian community, *Midwife, Health Visitor and Community Nurse*, 19(12): 471–3.
Chitty, L. and Winter, R.M. (1989) Perinatal mortality in different ethnic groups, *Archives of Disease in Childhood*, 64: 1036–41.
Clarke, M. and Clayton, D. (1983) Quality of obstetric care provided for Asian immigrants in Leicester, *British Medical Journal*, 286: 621–3.
Clarke, M., Clayton, D.G., Mason, E.S. and MacVicar, J. (1988) Asian mothers' risk factors for perinatal death – the same or different? A 10-year review of Leicestershire perinatal deaths, *British Medical Journal*, 297: 384–7.
Clarke, M., Samani, N. and Diamond, P. (1979) Tuberculosis mortality among immigrants, *Community Medicine*, 1: 23–8.
Cunningham, A.M. (1984) *Teenage Pregnancy: The Social Making and Un-making of Mothers*. Birmingham: Pepar Publications.
Currer, C. (1986) Concept of mental well- and ill-being: the case of Pathan mothers in Britain, in C. Currer and M. Stacey (eds) *Concept of Health and Illness and Disease*. Oxford: Berg.
Day, S. (1994) Women from the Indian subcontinent: attitudes to contraception among Asian women in Britain, *Professional Care of Mother and Child*: 66–9.
Dobson, S.M. (1988) Transcultural health visiting: caring in a multicultural society, *Recent Advances in Nursing*, 20: 61–80.
Donovan, J.L. (1983) Black people's health: a different way forward, *Radical Community Medicine*, Winter: 20–9.
Donovan, J.L. (1984) Ethnicity and health: a research review, *Social Science and Medicine*, 19(7): 663–70.
Donovan, J.L. (1986) *We Don't Buy Sickness, It Just Comes: Health, Illness and Health Care in the Lives of Black People in London*. Aldershot: Gower.
Drury, B. (1991) Sikh girls and the maintenance of an ethnic culture, *New Community*, 17(3): 387–99.
Dwyer, R. (1994) Caste, religion and sect in Gujarat, in R. Ballard (ed.) *Desh Pardesh: The South Asian Presence in Britain*. London: Hurst.
Eade, J. (1990) Bangladeshi community organisation and leadership in East London, in C. Clarke, C. Peach and S. Vertovec (eds) *South Asians Overseas*. Cambridge: Cambridge University Press.
Eade, J., Vamplew, T. and Peach, C. (1996) The Bangladeshis: the encapsulated community, in C. Peach (ed.) *Ethnicity in the 1991 Census, Volume Two: The Ethnic Minority Populations of Great Britain*. London: HMSO.
Edwards, J. (1994) *Multilingualism*. Harmondsworth: Penguin.
Eiser, C. and Eiser, R. (1985) Mothers' experience on the post-natal ward, *Child: care, health and development*, 13: 75–85.
Elbourne, D., Oakley, A. and Chalmers, I. (1989) Social and psychological support during pregnancy, in I. Chalmers, M. Enkin and M. Keirse (eds) *Effective Care in Pregnancy and Childbirth*, Vol. 1, Parts I–V. Oxford: Oxford University Press.

El-Islam, M.F., Malasi, T.H. and Abu-Dagga, S.I. (1988) Oral-contraceptives, socio-cultural beliefs and psychiatric symptoms, *Social Science and Medicine*, 27(9): 941–5.

Enkin, M. and Chalmers, I. (eds) (1982) *Effectiveness and Satisfaction in Antenatal Care*. London: William Heinemann Medical Books Ltd.

Enkin, M., Keirse, J. and Chalmers, I. (1990) *A Guide to Effective Care in Pregnancy and Childbirth*. Oxford: Oxford University Press.

Firdous, R. and Bhopal, R.S. (1989) Reproductive health of Asian women: a comparative study with hospital and community perspectives, *Public Health* 103: 307–15.

Fleissig, A. (1993) Are women given enough information by staff during labour and delivery?, *Midwifery*, 9: 70–5.

Foster, K., Lader, D. and Cheesbrough, S. (1997) *Infant Feeding 1995: Results from a Survey Carried out in England by the Social Survey Division of ONS on Behalf of the Department of Health*. London: The Stationery Office.

Garcia, J. (1982) Women's views of antenatal care, in M. Enkin and I. Chalmers (eds) (1982) *Effectiveness and Satisfaction in Antenatal Care*. London: William Heinemann Medical Books Ltd.

Garcia, J., Kilpatrick, R. and Richards, M. (eds) (1990) *The Politics of Maternity Care: Services for Childbearing Women in Twentieth-Century Britain*. Oxford: Clarendon Press.

Gillies, D.R.N., Lealman, G.T., Lumb, K.M. and Congdon, P. (1984) Analysis of ethnic influence on stillbirth and infant mortality in Bedford 1975–81, *Journal of Epidemiology and Community Health*, 38: 214–17.

Gladman, J. (1994) Antenatal care in the '90s, *British Journal of Midwifery*, 2(10): 449–503.

Goel, K.M., Campbell, S., Logan, R.W., Sweet, E.M., Attenborrow, A. and Arneil, G.C. (1981) Reduced prevalence of rickets in Asian children in Glasgow, *Lancet*, 2: 405–7.

Graham, H. (1977) Women's attitudes to conception and pregnancy, in R. Chester and J. Peel (eds) *Equality and Inequality in Family Life*. London: Academic Press.

Graham, H. and McKee, L. (1980) The First Months of Motherhood Vol. 1: Summary Report. Unpublished report, London: Health Education Council.

Graham, H. and Oakley, A. (1981) Competing ideologies of reproduction: medical and maternal perspectives on pregnancy, in H. Robert (ed.) *Women, Health and Reproduction*. London: Routledge and Kegan Paul.

Green, J.M. (1993) Expectations and experiences of pain in labour: findings from a large prospective study, *Birth*, 20(2): 65–72.

Green, J.M., Coupland, V.A. and Kitzinger, J.V. (1990) Expectations, experiences, and psychological outcomes of childbirth: a prospective study of 825 women, *Birth*, 17(1): 15–24.

Haines, A.P., McFadyen, I.R., Campbell-Brown, M., North, W.R.S. and Abraham, R. (1982) Birthweight and complications of pregnancy in an Asian population, in I. McFadyen, and J. MacVicar (eds) *Obstetric Problems of the Asian Community in Britain*. London: Royal College of Obstetricians and Gynaecologists.

Haire, D. (1978) The cultural warping of childbirth, in J. Ehrenreich (ed.) *The Cultural Crisis of Modern Medicine*. New York: Monthly Review Press.

HEA (Health Education Authority) (1994) *Black and Minority Ethnic Groups in England: Health and Lifestyles*. London: Health Education Authority.

Hern, W. (1971) Is pregnancy really normal?, *Family Planning Perspectives*, 3(1): 5–10.
Homans, H. (1980) Pregnant in Britain: a sociological approach to Asian and British women's experiences. Unpublished PhD Thesis, University of Warwick.
Homans, H. (1982) Pregnancy and birth as rites of passage for two groups of women in Britain, in C.P. MacCormack (ed.) *Ethnography of Fertility and Birth*. London: Academic Press.
Homans, H. (1983) A question of balance: Asian and British Women's perception of food during pregnancy, in A. Murcott (ed.) *The Sociology of Food and Eating*. London: Gower.
Homans, H. (1985a) (ed.) *The Sexual Politics of Reproduction*. Aldershot: Gower.
Homans, H. (1985b) Discomforts in pregnancy: traditional remedies and medical prescriptions, in H. Homans (ed.) *The Sexual Politics of Reproduction*. Aldershot: Gower.
Honeyman, M.M., Bahl, L., Marshall, T. and Wharton, B.A. (1987) Consanguinity and fetal growth in Pakistani Moslems, *Archives of Disease in Childhood*, 62: 231–5.
House of Commons Home Affairs Committee (1986) *Bangladeshi in Britain* (1st Report). London: HMSO.
Hussain, J. (1991) The Bengali speech community, in S. Allaldina and V. Edwards (eds) *Multilingualism in the British Isles*, Vol. 2. London: Longman.
Hussain, F. and Radwan, K. (1984) The Islamic revolution and women: quest for the Quranic model, in F. Hussain (ed.) *Muslim Women*. Kent: Croom Helm.
Illich, I. (1976) *Limits to Medicine, Medical Nemesis: The Expropriation of Health*. Harmondsworth: Penguin.
Inch, S. (1982) *Birthrights*. London: Hutchinson.
Jackson-Baker, A. (1988) Antenatal care: boon or bore, *Nursing Times*, 84: 69–70.
Jain, C. (1985) *Attitudes of Pregnant Asian Women to Antenatal Care*. Birmingham: West Midlands Regional Health Authority.
Jeffery, P., Jeffery, R. and Lyons, A. (1989) *Labour Pains and Labour Power: Women and Childbearing in India*. London: Zed Books.
Jordanova, L.J. (1980) Natural facts, in C. MacCormack and M. Strathern (eds) *Nature, Culture and Gender*. Cambridge: Cambridge University Press.
Kabeer, N. (1985) Do women gain from high fertility?, in H. Afshar (ed.) *Women, Work and Ideology in the Third World*. London: Tavistock.
Katbamna, S., Bhakta, P., Parker, G. and Ahmad, W.I.U. (1997) *The Needs of Asian Carers: A Selective Review of Literature*, WP50 11/96. Leicester: Nuffield Community Care Studies Unit, University of Leicester.
Katzner, K. (1977) *The Languages of the World*. London: Routledge and Kegan Paul.
Kearns, R.A., Neuwelt, P.M., Hitchman, B. and Lennan, M. (1997) Social support and psychological distress before and after childbirth, *Health and Social Care in the Community*, 5(5): 296–308.
Kitzinger, J. (1990) Strategies of the early childbirth movement: a case-study of the National Childbirth Trust, in J. Garcia, R. Kilpatrick and M. Richards (eds) *The Politics of Maternity Care: Services for Childbearing Women in Twentieth-Century Britain*. Oxford: Clarendon.
Kitzinger, S. (1962) *The Experience of Childbirth*. London: Gollancz.
Kitzinger, S. (1978) *Women as Mothers*. London: Fontana Books.
Kitzinger, S. (1987) *Some Women's Experience of Epidurals*. London: National Childbirth Trust.

Kitzinger, S. and Davis, J. (eds) (1978) *The Place of Birth*. Oxford: Oxford University Press.
Kitzinger, S. and Walter, A. (1981) *Some Women's Experience of Episiotomy*. London: National Childbirth Trust.
Koo, L.C. (1984) The use of food to treat and prevent disease in Chinese culture, *Social Science and Medicine*, 18(9): 757–66.
Leeds Family Health Services Authority (1992) *Research into the Uptake of Maternity Services as Provided by Primary Health Care Teams to Women from Black and Ethnic Minorities*. Leeds: Family Health Services Authority.
Lewis, P. (1994) Being Muslim and being British: the dynamics of Islamic reconstruction in Bradford, in R. Ballard (ed.) *Desh Pardesh: The South Asian Presence in Britain*. London: Hurst.
Liddle, J. and Joshi, R. (1986) *Daughters of Independence: Gender, Caste and Class in India*. London: Zed Books.
Littlewood, R. and Lipsedge, M. (1982) *Aliens and Alienists*. Harmondsworth: Penguin.
LMP (Linguistic Minorities Project) (1985) *The Other Languages of England*. London: Routledge.
Lone, R. (1987) Asian women and health, Women's Health Information Centre *Newsletter*, 7 (Spring).
Lozoff, B., Jordan, B. and Malone, S. (1988) Childbirth in cross-cultural perspective, *Marriage and Family Review*, 2: 35–60.
McAvoy, B.R. and Raza, R. (1988) Asian women: (i) Contraceptive knowledge, attitudes and usage, (ii) Contraceptive services and cervical cytology, *Health Trends*, 20: 11–17.
MacCarthy, B. and Craissati, J. (1989) Ethnic differences in response to adversity: a community sample of Bangladeshis and their indigenous neighbours, *Social Psychiatry and Psychiatric Epidemiology*, 24: 196–201.
MacCormack, C.P. (ed.) (1982) *Ethnography of Fertility and Birth*. London: Academic Press.
McDonald, M. (1987) Rituals of motherhood among Gujarati women in East London, in R. Burghardt (ed.) *Hinduism in Great Britain*. London: Tavistock.
McEnery, G. and Rao, K.P.S. (1986) The effectiveness of antenatal education of Pakistani and Indian women living in this country, *Child: care, health and development*, 12: 385–99.
MacFarlane, A. (1984) Facts, beliefs and misconceptions about the bonding process, in L. Zander and G. Chamberlain (eds) *Pregnancy Care for the 1980s*. London: Royal Society of Medicine and Macmillan.
MacIntyre, S. (1981) *The Expectations and Experiences of First Pregnancy*. Occasional Paper No. 5. University of Aberdeen, Institute of Medical Sociology.
McIntosh, J. (1989) Models of childbirth and social class: a study of 80 working-class primigravidae, in S. Robinson and A.M. Thomson (eds) *Midwives, Research and Childbirth, Vol. 1*. London: Chapman and Hall.
Mckinlay, J. (1972) The sick role – illness and pregnancy, *Social Science and Medicine*, 6: 561–72.
Mayor, V. (1984) The Asian community, pregnancy, childbirth and childcare, *Nursing Times*, 80(24): 57–8.
Messenger-Davies, M. (1986) *The Breastfeeding Book*. London: Century.
Messer, E. (1981) Hot–cold classification: theoretical and practical implications of a Mexican study, *Social Science and Medicine*, 15B: 133–45.

Modood, T., Berthoud, R., Lakey, J., Nazroo, J., Smith, P., Virdee, S. and Belshon, S. (1997) *Ethnic Minorities in Britain: Diversity and Disadvantage*. London: Policy Studies Institute.

MORI (1993) *East London Health: Research Study Conducted for City and East London FHSA*. London: MORI.

Moss, P., Bolland, G., Foxman, R. and Owen, C. (1987) The hospital inpatient stay: the experience of first-time parents, *Child: care, health and development*, 13: 153–67.

Narang, I. and Murphy, S. (1994) Assessment of antenatal care for Asian women, *British Journal of Midwifery*, 2(4): 169–73.

NCT (National Childbirth Trust) (1992) *Pregnancy, Birth and Parenthood*. Oxford: Oxford University Press.

NHS/CRD (1996) *A Pilot Study of 'Informed Choice' Leaflets on Positions in Labour and Routine Ultrasound*. University of York: NHS Center for Review and Disseminations.

Niven, C.A. (1992) *Psychological Care for Families: before, during and after Birth*. London: Butterworth-Heinemann.

Oakley, A. (1976) Wisewoman and medicine man: changes in the management of childbirth, in J. Mitchell and A. Oakley (eds) *The Rights and Wrongs of Women*. Harmondsworth: Penguin.

Oakley, A. (1977) Cross-cultural practices, in T. Chard and M. Richards (eds) *Benefits and Hazards of the New Obstetrics*. London: Heinemann Medical Books.

Oakley, A. (1979) *Becoming a Mother*. Oxford: Martin Robertson.

Oakley, A. (1980) *Women Confined: Towards a Sociology of Childbirth*. Oxford: Martin Robertson.

Oakley, A. (1981) *Subject Women*. Oxford: Martin Robertson.

Oakley, A. (1984) *The Captured Womb: a history of the medical care of pregnant women*. Oxford: Blackwell.

Oakley, A. (1992) *Social Support and Motherhood: The Natural History of a Research Project*. Oxford: Blackwell.

Oakley, A. and Richards, M. (1990) Women's experiences of Caesarean delivery, in J. Garcia, R. Kilpatrick and M. Richards (eds) *The Politics of Maternity Care: Services for Childbearing Women in Twentieth-Century Britain*. Oxford: Clarendon.

OPCS (1991) *Country of Birth and Ethnic Group Report*. London: HMSO.

Owen, D. (1994) *South Asian People in Great Britain: Social and Economic Circumstances*, 1991 Census Statistical Paper No. 7, University of Warwick.

Parsons, L. and Day, S. (1992) Improving obstetric outcomes in ethnic minorities: an evaluation of health advocacy in Hackney, *Journal of Public Health Medicine*, 14(2): 183–91.

Parsons, L., Macfarlane, A. and Golding, J. (1993) Pregnancy, birth and maternity care, in W.I.U. Ahmad (ed.) *'Race' and Health in Contemporary Britian*. Buckingham: Open University Press.

Pearson, M. (1983) The politics of ethnic minority health studies, *Radical Community Medicine*, Winter: 34–44.

Pearson, M. (1986) Racist notions of ethnicity and culture in health education, in S. Rodmell and A. Watt (eds) *The Politics of Health Education*. London: Tavistock.

Pearson, M. (1991) Ethnic differences in infant health, *Archives of Disease in Childhood*, 66: 88–90.

Perkins, E.R. (1980) *Men on the Labour Ward*. Leverhulme Health Education Project, Occasional Paper No. 22. Nottingham: University of Nottingham.

Pharoah, P.O.D. and Alberman, E.D. (1990) Annual Statistical Review, *Archives of Disease in Childhood*, 65: 147–51.

Phillips, K. (1985) Asians in Britain, *Midwife, Health Visitor and Community Nurse*, 21: 114–18.

Phoenix, A. (1990a) Black women and the maternity services, in J. Garcia, R. Kilpatrick and M. Richards (eds) *The Politics of Maternity Care: Services for Childbearing Women in Twentieth-Century Britain*. Oxford: Clarendon.

Phoenix, A. (1990b) *Young Mothers?* Oxford: Polity Press.

Phoenix, A., Woollett, A. and Lloyd, E. (eds) (1991) *Motherhood: Meanings, Practices and Ideologies*. London: Sage.

Pillsbury, B.L.K. (1978) 'Doing the month': confinement and convalescence of Chinese women after childbirth, *Social Science and Medicine*, 12: 11–22.

Rack, P. (1980) *Race, Culture and Mental Disorder*. London: Tavistock.

Rashid, J. (1983) Contraceptive use among Asian women, *British Journal of Family Planning*, 8: 132–5.

Raja, V. (1993) Conceptions of health and health care among two generations of Gujarati-speaking Hindu women in Leicester. Unpublished MPhil Thesis, Department of Sociology, University of Leicester.

Reid, M. (1990) Pre-natal diagnosis and screening: a review, in J. Garcia, R. Kilpatrick and M. Richards (eds) *The Politics of Maternity Care: Services for Childbearing Women in Twentieth-Century Britain*. Oxford: Clarendon.

Richardson, D. (1993) *Women, Motherhood and Childrearing*. Basingstoke: Macmillan.

Robinson, S. (1990) Maintaining the independence of the midwifery profession: a continuing struggle, in J. Garcia, R. Kilpatrick and M. Richards (eds) *The Politics of Maternity Care: Services for Childbearing Women in Twentieth-Century Britain*. Oxford: Clarendon.

Robinson, V. (1996) The Indians: onward and upward, in C. Peach (ed.) *Ethnicity in the 1991 Census, Vol. 2: The Ethnic Minority Populations of Great Britain*. London: HMSO.

Rocheron, Y. (1988) The Asian Mother and Baby Campaign: the construction of ethnic minorities' health needs, *Critical Social Policy*, 22: 4–23.

Rocheron, Y. and Dickinson, R. (1990) The Asian Mother and Baby Campaign: a way forward in health promotion for Asian women? *Health Education Journal*, 49(3): 128–33.

Rocheron, Y., Dickinson, R. and Khan, S. (1989) *The Evaluation of the Asian Mother and Baby Campaign: Full Summary*. Leicester: Centre for Mass Communication Research, University of Leicester.

Runnymede Trust and Radical Statistics Group (1980) *Britain's Black Population*. London: Heinemann Educational Books.

Rush, D. (1982) Effects of changes in protein and calorie intake during pregnancy on the growth of the human fetus, in M. Enkin and I. Chalmers (eds) *Effectiveness and Satisfaction in Antenatal Care*. London: William Heinemann Medical Books Ltd.

Schott, J. and Henley, A. (1996) *Culture, Religion and Childbearing in a Multiracial Society: A Handbook for Health Professionals*. Oxford: Butterworth-Heinemann.

Sen, D. and Holmes, C. (1996) Newcastle Bangladeshi Midwifery Project, *MIDIRS Midwifery Digest*, 6(2): 225–9.

Sheilham, H. and Quick, A. (1982) *The Rickets Report*. London: Haringey Community Health Council and Community Relations Council.
Sheldon, T. and Parker, H. (1992) Use of 'ethnicity' and race in health research: a cautionary note, in W.I.U. Ahmad (ed.) *The Politics of 'Race' and Health*. Bradford: Race Relations Research Unit, University of Bradford, and Bradford and Ilkley Community College.
Simkin, P. and Enkin, M. (1989) Antenatal classes, in M. Enkin, J. Keirse and I. Chalmers, *A Guide to Effective Care in Pregnancy and Childbirth*. Oxford: Oxford University Press.
Smaje, C. (1995) *Health, 'Race' and Ethnicity: Making Sense of the Evidence*. London: Kings Fund Institute.
Spiro, A. (1994) Breastfeeding experiences of Gujarati women living in Harrow. Unpublished MSc Medical Anthropology Disseration, Brunel University.
Stacey, M. (1988) *The Sociology of Health and Healing*. London: Unwin Hyman.
Steer, P. (1993) Rituals in antenatal care – do we need them? *British Medical Journal*, 307: 697–8.
Stonham, K. and Sims, P. (1986) Asian women having babies in Luton, 1983: a controlled study, *Health and Hygiene*, 7: 10–12.
Stopes-Roe, M. and Cochrane, R. (1990) *Citizens of This Country: The Asian-British*. Clevedon: Multilingual Matters.
Stubbs, P. (1993) 'Ethnically sensitive' or 'anti-racist'? Models of health research and service delivery, in W.I.U. Ahmad (ed.) *'Race' and Health in Contemporary Britain*. Buckingham: Open University Press.
Swan, C. and Cooke, W. (1971) Nutritional Osteomalacia in Immigrants, *Lancet*, 2(i): 456–9.
Tew, M. (1990) *Safer Childbirth? A Critical History of Maternity Care*. London: Chapman and Hall.
Theodore-Gandi, B. and Shaikh, K. (1988) *Maternity Services Consumers Survey Report*. Bradford: Bradford Health Authority.
Thomas, M. and Avery, V. (1997) *Infant Feeding in Asian Families: A Survey Carried Out in England by the Social Survey Division of ONS on Behalf of the Department of Health*. London: The Stationery Office.
Thompson, C. (1985) The power to pollute and the power to preserve: perceptions of female power in a Hindu village, *Social Science and Medicine*, 21(6): 701–11.
Thomson, A.M. (1989) Why don't women breast feed?, in S. Robinson and A.M. Thomson (eds) *Midwives, Research and Childbirth, Vol. 1*. London: Chapman and Hall.
Tones, B.K. (1981) The use and abuse of mass media in health education, in D.S. Leather, G.B. Hasting and J.K. Davies (eds) *Health Education and the Media*. Oxford: Pergamon Press.
Townsend, S. and Davidson, N. (1982) *Inequalities in Health: The Black Report*. Harmondsworth: Penguin.
Trivedi, A. (1920) Terms of relationship among the Gujarati Hindus, *Indian Journal of Sociology*, 1(3): 274–84.
Versluysen, M.C. (1981) Midwives, medical men and 'poor women labouring of child': lying-in hospitals in eighteenth-century London, in H. Roberts (ed.) *Women, Health and Reproduction*. London: Routledge and Kegan Paul.
Visram, R. (1986) *Ayahs, Lascars and Princes: Indians in Britain 1700–1947*. London: Pluto Press.

Walvin, J. (1984) *Passage to Britain*. Harmondsworth: Pelican.
Westwood, S. and Bhachu, P. (1988) (eds) *Enterprising Women: Economy and Gender Relations*. London: Routledge.
Westwood, S., Couloute, J., Desai, S., Matthew, P. and Piper, A. (1989) *Sadness in My Heart: Racism and Mental Health*. Leicester: Leicester Black Mental Health Group, University of Leicester.
Wharton, B. (1982) Food, growth and the Asian fetus, in I. McFadyen and J. MacVicar (eds) *Obstetric Problems of the Asian Community in Britain*. London: Royal College of Obstetricians and Gynaecologists.
Whitehead, M. (1992) *The Health Divide*, revised edn., Harmondsworth: Penguin.
Windsor-Richards, K. and Gillies, P.A. (1988) Racial grouping and women's experiences of giving birth in hospital, *Midwifery*, 4: 171–6.
Wolkind, S. and Zajicek, E. (1981) *Pregnancy: A Psychological and Social Study*. London: Academic Press.
Woollett, A. and Dosanjh-Matwala, N. (1990a) Pregnancy and antenatal care: the attitudes and experiences of Asian women, *Child: care, health and development*, 16: 63–78.
Woollett, A. and Dosanjh-Matwala, N. (1990b) Postnatal care: the attitudes and experiences of Asian women in east London, *Midwifery*, 6: 178–84.
Woollett, A., Dosanjh-Matwala, N. and Hadlow, J. (1991) The attitudes to contraception of Asian women in East London, *British Journal of Family Planning*, 17: 72–7.
Woollett, A., Dosanjh, N., Nicolson, P., Marshall, H., Djhanbakhch, O. and Hadlow, J. (1995) The ideas and experiences of pregnancy and childbirth of Asian and non-Asian women in East London, *British Journal of Medical Psychology*, 68: 65–84.
Worthington-Roberts, B. and Williams, S.R. (1993) *Nutrition in Pregnancy and Lactation*, 5th edn. St. Louis, MO: Mosby.
Zaida, F. (1994) The maternity care of Muslim women, *Professional Midwife*, 4(3): 8–10.
Zaklama, M. (1984) The Asian community in Leicester and the family planning services, *Biology and Society*, 1: 63–9.
Zola, I.K. (1978) Medicine as an institution of social control, in J. Ehrenreich (ed.) *The Cultural Crisis of Modern Medicine*. New York: Monthly Review Press.

# Index